What Reviewers Are Sa
ALL-TERRAIN SKIING II

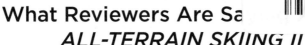

"*All-Terrain Skiing II* will revolutionize instructional ski books. In fact, calling this an instructional book seems like the wrong label. Maybe *The Skiing Scriptures* will do. Or perhaps *The Tao of Downhill*."

Mike Finkel, Author and former Skiing magazine contributing editor

"For more than ten years, skiers from all over the globe have been coming to Big Sky Resort for Dan Egan's Steeps Camps. His unique teaching style keeps guests coming back year after year to ski Big Sky's most iconic runs with Dan. We're thrilled to have Dan call Big Sky home each winter."

Christine Baker, Vice President of Mountain Sports, Big Sky Resort

"Steeps Camp with Dan Egan was one of the ultimate experiences I have had in my decades of skiing. Dan and his team did a great job meeting people where they were, and no one felt pushed to do anything they did not want to do. I have always loved steep terrain, and I fell in love with Big Sky. The Steeps Camp was transformative, and I will return!"

Matt Mandel, California

"Wow, three days of learning and great skiing. The time and thought Dan has invested in the curriculum, the insights, the coaching, and even the logistics was readily apparent, and I'm grateful for his willingness to pass his experience and excitement on to others. It's a great program, and I'm happy to share that with anyone who'll listen!"

Jonathan Bryant

"I've taken clinics with Dan throughout North America, Europe, and New Zealand. Thanks to him, I finally broke out of my skiing rut."

Eric Foch, Park City, UT

"For the past twelve years, I have been on the Big Sky Snow Sports staff and have had the pleasure of watching and participating in clinics coached by Dan Egan. When I am asked by my clientele about skiing some of the steep terrain on Lone Peak, I always recommend they attend Dan's Steeps Camp or engage a Mountain Guide who has been trained by Dan. In fact, when I hear the word 'steep,' I see Dan in my mind's eye!"

Mike Ewing
PSIA Certified Instructor for 58 years.
Author of *My life In Winters*

ALL-TERRAIN SKIING II

ALL-TERRAIN SKIING II
Body Mechanics and Balance, from Powder to Ice

Instruction * Drills * Exercises

Dan Egan

Degan Media, Inc.
Campton, NH

Published by Degan Media Inc.

Paperback ISBN-13: 978-1-7364927-7-2

First paperback edition October 2022

Book design: Eddie Vincent, ENC Graphic Services
Cover design by Christopher Wait and Deirdre Wait, ENC Graphic Services
Front Cover Photograph: Warren Miller Entertainment, Ian Anderson
Back Cover Photos: Jen Bennett, Rumble Productions; Mike McPhee; and Bob Legassa, Freeride Media
Author Photograph by Kathryn Costello Photography

Edited by: Jack Rochester Joshua Tree Interactive and Courtney Jenkins Soaring Arrow Editing

ATS App Design: Jasper Ladkin & CK Padayao
Video for the App, shot on location in Laax Switzerland and Big Sky, MT
Video Shot by: Tom Day, Patti Johnson, Chris Kamman, Satchele Burns
Video Edited by: Corey Potter, Chief Productions
Images of Drills shot by Tom Day, Patti Johnson & Chris Kamman

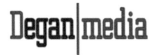

Published by Degan Media, Inc.
PO Box #988, Campton, NH, 03233
www.Dan-Egan.com
www.Skiclinics.com

Dedicated to
My Parents,
Mary Ellen Gillis "Marlen" and Robert W. Egan

TABLE OF CONTENTS

ORIGINAL FOREWORD FROM
ALL-TERRAIN SKIING I

IN MY TWENTY-FIVE YEARS AS a skier, and nearly a decade as an editor of *Skiing* magazine, I have worked out a highly specialized system of classifying top-notch skiers. There are expert skiers, extreme skiers, ski bums, ski starts, ski instructors, ski pros—and then there is Dan Egan.

Dan is the most dedicated, most spirited, most head-over-heels-in-love-with-sliding-on-snow skier I have ever encountered. He eats skiing; he breathes skiing; hell, he sweats skiing. He has traveled the world preaching the gospel of skiing—a one-man mogul-skiing missionary—the Johnny Appleseed of face-shots. His movies, which always bring to life the cultures and ski scenes of unimaginable lands, are the skiing equivalent of a National Geographic special. I have never met anyone quite like him. Dan is so far beyond normal classifications of skiers that there was no choice but to grant him a category all to himself.

I was first introduced to Dan as a student in one of his clinics, at a small Vermont ski area called Bolton Valley. I was immediately struck by his unique insights, his effortless humor, and his endearing eccentricity. His energy is unparalleled: a ski lesson with Dan is part Einstein, part Freud, and part Groucho Marx. "A full-soul approach to skiing," I call it. A dozen of his personalized pointers—one about edging on ice, another about absorbing moguls, a third about maintaining a quiet upper body (and several of his bad jokes)— remain with me to recall when I'm having an off day on the slopes.

I have skied with him several times since, and his unflagging enthusiasm has never failed to fill me with joy. I have always had the impression that life, for Dan, is a perpetual powder day. To take a few runs with him is always a season highlight, no matter the ski conditions.

I've been waiting years for Dan to write a book like this, so that his unusual ideas are readily accessible to all skiers. In quintessential Dan—clear, concise, and bizarre—*All-Terrain Skiing* will revolutionize the instructional ski book. In fact, calling this an instructional book would be the wrong label. Maybe *The Skiing Scriptures* will do. Or perhaps *The Tao of Downhill*. Only a book cooked by Dan could have drills called Mind Over Mogul and The Joy of Skiing. Only a book by Dan would ask you to take your skis off and walk down the hill. Only Dan will ask you to flap your arms as you ski, or clap your hands, or ski with your boots unbuckled. There is material in here to help and amuse and enlighten every skier at every level.

So, stifle your inhibitions, drop your doubts, and open your mind. Read this book, study it, bring the cards on the chairlift. Ease into Dan's world. Laugh at the tales of his crazy adventures and discover a whole new way to improve your skiing.

Mike Finkel
Bozeman, Montana

INTRODUCTION TO THE SECOND EDITION

IT'S AMAZING TO THINK ABOUT releasing *All-Terrain Skiing* in 1996, as the world was very different then, in both technology and in sport. We were just starting to produce DVDs instead of VHS tapes. Ski companies were beginning to introduce the idea of shaped, wider skis. As a matter of fact, we didn't even address carving, shaped, or powder skis in the original version of this book. I did write an article for *Skiing* magazine that year, titled "[The] Lost Art of Skiing," which spoke to the many movements of skiing that would disappear with the advent of new ski shapes. For the most part, that has proven to be true.

Today, with the new wider, shaped skis, we can glide right over the snow. In the straight-ski days, we plowed through the snow and needed a lot of momentum in order to pump the skis up and down. We also had to make many more turns than we do today. When people watch the old films, they always comment on how many turns we made while skiing a chute or a wide-open powder field. However, as the adage goes, the more things change the more they stay the same, and for most ski techniques that has remained true.

What I see in many of the skiers who take my camps and clinics is how they rely too much on the equipment to do the work, and not enough on body mechanics. This results in fatigue and an overall lack of balance in varying conditions and challenging terrain. And without practice a skier lacks speed control, or over-controls their speed. Either way, the skier lacks the confidence to let their skis run and flow.

As a result, I still teach many of the skills and drills found in the first edition of *All-Terrain Skiing* because they refocus the energy on inherent body movements, rather than steering or skidding the ski. The body mechanics outlined in this book help skiers as they encounter changes in speed, terrain, conditions, and situations.

The *All-Terrain Skiing* program is organized into five categories: Balance, Upper Body, Power, Fluidity, and Agility, with individual drills described in each chapter. These drills help you make body alignments while in motion, which ultimately increases your efficiency of motion and allows you to ski longer and with more control.

In the Introduction to the first edition of *All-Terrain Skiing*, I stated, "I was never too cool for ski school. Nevertheless, I was exposed to ski lessons from the time I was five until I was seventeen. Every winter Saturday, my siblings and I would jump on a bus and head north to ski country with the Blizzard Ski Club." And years later, during an interview with *Skiing* magazine, the writer asked, "How did a kid from a suburb of Boston grow up to become one of the top extreme skiers in the world?" At that moment, I realized the importance of ski schools. All those Saturday lessons and the basic ski techniques taught by competent ski instructors, combined with a powerful desire to become the best at whatever I set my mind to, made me the skier I am today.

In this book, you'll learn thirty-one ski drills designed to make you a better, more efficient skier. Skiers who take my camps and clinics always mention how the drills instilled a new freedom of movement into their skiing. The goal is to develop a new awareness of your relationship to gravity in a variety of ski conditions, to dynamically orient and angulate your body to maximize control and efficiency, and to achieve constant, fluid motion.

Skiing is not an intellectual activity; skiing is a simple physical activity based on good body position.

Keep these four principles in mind, and you'll soon be skiing better than ever:

- **Good balance**
- **Powerful stance with shoulders square to the hill**
- **Eyes focused up or down the hill**
- **Proper hand position**

The goal of this book is for you to become aware of every aspect of your body positioning in order to expand where and how you ski the mountain. The drills are designed to take your mind off performance and focus your body energy on the task at hand. By removing the projected outcome, we can zero in on how to react in each moment to changing situations, terrain, and conditions. This will enhance our performance overall.

Every skier should begin with Balance before progressing in order through Upper Body, Power, Fluidity, and Agility. Assess your skills and your skill level, then work on mastering one set of drills at a time. Each drill complements every other drill, building competence. Even if some of the drills seem silly or simple at first, as you practice you'll see how they progressively require more energy. And as your program builds, so will your confidence and courage to try high-end maneuvers.

In my new book, *Mastering the Skiing Mind*, which will be released in Fall of 2023, I will further develop the ideas and concepts of efficient body movements while skiing free of judgement and allowing skiers and riders to enter the "flow state," free from the negative mind.

First, master the drills in this book. They will help you develop skills which can help you ski from powder to ice, groomed slopes to steep slopes, and beyond. The drills in this book are specifically designed to create a powerful, athletic ski stance for skiers of all abilities.

There are lots of "skiing gurus" and professional ski instructors who have developed specific teaching techniques to help skiers improve. Some will tell you carving is the ultimate skill. Others will say that edge angle matters. And still others focus on knees, hips, and hands. I will introduce you to a wide range of body motions and skills through drills that simply ask you to be calm and strong, fluid and loose. Learning to do this will increase your balance as you move downhill over varying terrain.

My simple goal is to help earnest skiers improve by concentrating first and primarily on their mental state and body:

Mind. Most skiers don't understand the importance of being mentally prepared, as well as physically in shape, to ski. I begin with an understanding of the human mind and body, exploring desire, confidence, and will power.

Body. I'm always amazed to see skiers who rise, drink a cup of coffee, then head up the slopes and wonder why they have burning thighs by ten o'clock. Here, we focus on breathing to provide the oxygen muscles need to perform well. Our goal is to increase your efficiency.

Equipment. With today's equipment, confusion can arise when shopping for the right boots, ski length and ski width, and other selling features. I will provide some basic guidance based on simplicity, cost, and skill level.

Conditions. One thing is certain—the skier will always encounter changing (if not challenging) terrain and conditions. The *All-Terrain Skiing* program teaches the progressive skiing skills needed for everything from groomed trails to deep powder.

All-Terrain Skiing II is an integrated, self-contained program for beginning, intermediate, and advanced skiers—in other words, anyone who wants to ski better. This book is organized for progressive learning. At the heart of the program are the thirty-one illustrated drills described in this book, along with a downloadable version, the ATS App, which you can install on your mobile phone for ready reference and practice on the slopes.

Lessons are identified with international trail marking symbols: Green Circle for beginners, Blue Square for intermediate, and Black Diamond for expert. In the ATS II App, they are also categorized by color—red for Balance, mauve for Upper Body, green for Power, blue for Fluidity, and gray for Agility—to help you organize your lessons for quick access. At the end of this book, as well as throughout, are articles I've written for "Explore Big Sky," the Montana newspaper and website. These articles complement and expand on the concepts, drills, and skills in this book.

FREEDOM FOUND IN SKIING

THE FREEDOM FOUND IN SKIING and snowboarding is instant and rewarding. From the moment you point yourself downhill, gravity takes over. Going with the flow is often the best decision. I like to say, "Don't let a bad turn contaminate the next good one." With that in mind, my goal setting is always focused forward, remembering that the achievement is a subset of the whole.

My suggested plan is always to start small and work up to the big stuff, which is how this book is laid out. To reiterate so you won't forget—this is a simple program based on balance, upper body position, power and/or dynamic motion, fluidity, and agility. It is designed for skiers of any ability to follow and learn how to improve.

In the mountains, surrounded by kindred spirits, I find my energy. When I ride up the lift and watch people gliding down the slope, something inside of me recognizes the connection others are having to this energy, and I sit in anticipation of it. Once I'm at the top and released from the lift, I join this force. I'm anchored by the Earth's gravitational pull. My eyes search out the fall line and I take a deep breath, then exhale, and push off. Now, in the first turn, the force and I are joined and I'm in this moment, free of the past. The world is forgotten. I'm at peace. It is so simple, so much fun, and so rewarding.

Skiers and riders often tell me about their aspirations—they've purchased new gear, gotten in shape, been praying for snow, and are committed to new challenges both large and small. Some are going to take a lesson, others go with a guide and accept that there will be risks. Often, they have a "bucket list" of runs and routes they hope to check off. These conversations are exciting, contagious, and easy to feed off of.

I often ask, "What is holding you back from doing these amazing things?" The answers tend to go across the board: not enough time or someone to do it with, a lack of experience, conditions haven't been right, recovering from an injury, last time they tried and fell, or someone told them they weren't ready. To sum it up in general terms, it's the "I cant's" and the "Ya-buts" that keep us from accomplishing goals. They bind us to a foundational fear, most often anchored in some way to the past.

I've never had such a list, yet I've gone to some amazing locations, stood on many a mountaintop, gazed at the surrounding beauty, and dropped down some jaw-dropping routes. Over the years I've found that to *find* a way, you must *enter into* what Taoism calls "The Way." As the ancient Chinese proverb goes, a journey of a thousand miles begins with a single step. This always reminds me to move forward, while striving to be free from the past. The pace of achievement is not important here; moving confidently into the future is. With each pole plant, turn, or run, I move away from the "Ya-buts" and the "I cant's" and enter into "The Way" of doing. I stay connected to the gravitational pull of the moment's challenge, moving toward a successful future.

1

Every day can be a fresh canvas, full of possibilities. It is often fueled by how we see it and to what we attach ourselves. Let this revised, updated, *All-Terrain Skiing II* program inspire your season of change. Commit to it; do the drills, master the skills, and you will see results as you journey through the process, moment by moment. Set your intention to moving forward one turn, one pole plant, one run at a time. Embrace learning new balance positions, edging skills, and body conditioning. Over time, your skiing will become more efficient and enjoyable. You'll be out on the mountain longer, skiing slopes and conditions you had only dreamed about.

THE GOLDEN RULE OF SKIING

THE GOLDEN RULE OF SKIING is: Ski the mountain, don't let the mountain ski you. To become a master of the mountain, you must learn to adapt to changing terrain and conditions while managing your speed. Always remember that you are the boss. Changes in terrain, conditions, and speed will expose flaws in any skier's technique. Skiing is a constant realignment of balance. Teach yourself to constantly deal with changing terrain and to trust your current ability in order to progress.

Find your own pace. Start by skiing at a constant speed, no matter the conditions. It is important to establish a skiing speed that is right for you. Speed should be determined by your ability to stop at any given moment. A good mogul skier, even after taking air, can stop on a dime. A racer skiing a slalom course must possess the ability to change direction at any moment, or else miss a gate.

Freeskiing the mountain is no different. Find a pace that feels comfortable to you. Begin and end your ski run at the same speed. Always make sure your first and last turns are the best. The first turn will set up your confidence and rhythm for the ensuing set of turns. Making your last turn the best is an insurance policy against injury caused by fatigue or carelessness. Using this rule, you'll find it easier to ski at a constant speed, which will give you more control.

Once you can ski at a constant speed, begin changing how you ski different terrain. Ski directly into a trail without stopping at the top. If you need to stop, pick a spot fifteen to twenty yards into the trail. This will provide an excellent opportunity for learning to adapt speed and technique to changing terrain. Discover the magic of entering a trail without stopping, instead turning and absorbing a knoll. Skiing into and through an intersection in complete control will turn heads as you fly away on the wide-open slope.

Make skiing fun by challenging yourself. For example, get off the lift ready to ski—boots buckled, helmet and poles strapped on—and head right off the lift and down your favorite trail. See how many turns you can make in a particular section of trail, or try making fifty turns all at the same radius and speed. Use the terrain to mix up slalom and giant slalom turns. Remind yourself that it's your mountain, you rule the school, and anything goes if you so deem it!

One of my favorite drills is nonstop skiing, top to bottom. Doing this a few times daily gets my adrenaline pumping. Skiing over changing terrain, adapting while in motion, is the best way to train your mind and body. Nothing can replace the experience of recovering your balance without stopping, making two sweeping turns around a corner, or skiing the fall line nonstop through the bumps. Mountains become less intimidating, and skiers begin to understand the fall lines and conditions of various trails, so small trouble spots pass by without a second thought and, more importantly, their new abilities enhance their confidence. Skiers who adapt to changing terrain, conditions, and speed will enjoy more of what the mountain has to offer. You will find yourself skiing terrain you never thought possible.

SPEED CONTROL IN THE WORLD OF NEW SKI PROFILE DESIGNS

THE ONLY PROFILE SKIS HAD for many years was turned up tip, camber and sidecut. But, since I wrote *All-Terrain Skiing* in 1995, ski design has changed—often. Most recently we have seen the introduction of *early rise* tips and *rockered* skis. When it comes to speed control, you want to be centered, and that is what these skis are all about. First, let's discuss what these terms mean and what the designs allow skiers to do, then talk about how they help control speed.

Skis have always had *camber*, a slight bowing in the center. Early rise skis may or may not have this camber beneath the foot. When choosing a profile, first ask yourself what percentage of groomed-slope skiing you do. If it's forty percent or greater, a ski with more camber might be best for you. Cambered skis provide more grip because the ski naturally flexes in the middle of the turn, then unflexes at the end, causing the edges to bite into the snow and thus provide a bit more grip, like a traditionally shaped ski.

Early rise skis, without that center camber under the foot, still edge well on groomed trails, but they also perform better in the woods and deeper snow because you can pivot more easily.

Rockered skis are often best for skiers who ski on groomed snow twenty percent or less of the time. These skis are designed to float in deeper snow and provide more stability at higher speeds than "fat" skis with camber.

Here is the key: Your skis want to tip and grip, and the sweet spot is in the center. On a traditional shaped ski, we can ski with a bit more forward-and-aft motion. But, since the tips and tails are pre-bent fore and aft on the newer skis, motion can create instability. To gain stability, you must stand solidly in the center of the skis, create an edge angle, and ride the arc. This creates the controllable acceleration you desire with little or no fore-and-aft movement.

The main benefit these new profiles provide is in their predetermined shape, which takes less body movement and energy to initiate a turn once the ski is on edge. Although each ski is designed slightly differently, they all share a common profile design: their tips and tails are pre-bent in the arc of a turn. Plus, a ski with no camber (flat under the foot), or a ski with reverse camber (tips and tails bent upwards just before and after the boot), will pivot or skid easier. This is helpful when skiing groomed slopes.

Traditionally shaped skis allow us to edge early in the turn, decelerate through edge pressure, then initiate the next turn. To accomplish this, you need to create pressure on the edge early in the arc, which is initiated through pressuring the tip. For many skiers, this was more easily accomplished with a shorter ski, which in turn led to shaped skis. Now, with these new designs, skis are growing longer again. With the early rise tip, we need more ski in front of the binding for grip, whether or not the ski is cambered.

With the new reverse camber and early rise skis, the sweet (balance) spot on hardpack snow is smaller. In deeper snow, the sweet spot is larger because the softer snow supports the arc of the ski. If you adjust your balance points on these newer skis, you'll soon grow to love them. Remember that solid ski technique remains the same, and a centered stance is the key to controlling your speed.

LEAN FORWARD

WHAT HAPPENED TO STANDING TALL when we ski? And why have most ski schools stopped teaching it? Years ago, the explanation I got from a nationally recognized ski instructor was, "We want skiers to move 'through' the turn in the transition, rather than 'up.'" I responded, "Don't we need to teach 'up' before we teach 'moving through in the transition?' Otherwise, how will skiers understand the feeling and the motion?" The response was, "Why teach something, then un-teach it?" My answer: "Because it is part of the progression of learning." In the end, we did not agree.

This is the crux of the problem with ski instruction today. We've refined it too much, and moved to a minimum-movement model rather than an exaggerated-motion model. Call me old school if you want, but I still focus on creating situations for skiers to explore motion and see how it affects the turning ski. Over time, once the movement is understood and mastered, it can be refined. That is the model I have had the most success with over the past thirty-five years.

So, let's dive in. The most overused saying in ski instruction is, "Lean forward and put pressure on the front of your boots." Even though this phrase is used by most ski instructors and coaches, many skiers ski sitting back, with more pressure over the tails of their skis rather than on the tips. Why?

It's a multi-part answer, and much of the confusion is over bending the knees. However, before we launch into solving this problem, let's explore the dynamics of how a ski works when we apply pressure to it.

There are three major sections of a ski.

> **Tip:** from the front end of the ski to three to four inches in front of the toe of the binding.
> **Midsection:** from three to four inches in front of the toe of the binding to three to four inches behind the heel of the binding.
> **Tail:** from three to four inches behind the heel of the binding to the end of the ski.

The previous lesson, "Speed Control in the World of New Ski Profile Designs," reviewed the new shapes of skis and how they perform. In this lesson, we will explore how applying pressure to the three main sections of the ski affects your turn.

When we put pressure on the tip of the ski, several things are accomplished, most importantly, this flexes the front section of the ski, which flexes the tip, initiating the turn—this is critical for controlling speed. A flexed ski absorbs energy.

If you only pressure the midsection of a ski without bending the tip, the ski tends to scoot forward, and instantly puts pressure on the tail—pressuring the tail is pure acceleration—and the combination of these two things moves your foot in front of your hip. And you lose control.

Many intermediate, and some expert skiers ski the midsection of the ski with little tip pressure very successfully in most conditions. Usually bumps, steeps, and narrow places will cause problems for skiers in this stance. But, in open spaces, they can cruise along feeling confident and having fun. However, eventually they will run into issues from being too far back on their ski. They can manage through athleticism, creating good angles, and keeping arms and shoulders over and in front of their feet. However, their hips are aft of their feet all the time.

Skiers who "sit back" generally pivot their skis to turn by twisting their feet rather than by carving turns. When hips, hands, and shoulders are aft of your feet, you have few options for turning, so you throw your hips into the turn and/or pivot your feet. This is a very limited way to achieve turning a ski. Here, too, skiers can have a wide range of success, but typically will avoid certain conditions and situations. If your weight is on your heels the result will be too much tail pressure, which creates unwanted acceleration.

The telltale sign of how people are standing on their skis and whether there is tip pressure is to watch the spray of the snow coming off their skis.

If there is an even flow of snow coming from two to six inches back from the tip throughout the entire ski during the turn, with no major bursts of spray at the end of the turn, there is consistent pressure on the ski through the entire turn.

If the snow spray starts in the midsection of the ski, the skier is in a neutral position, which will result in the ski scooting forward in the lower third of the turn. The skier will have to make some sort of bracing motion to slow ski. When there is a big burst of snow from the heel of the binding back, there is tail pressure. This causes skiers to develop inefficient movement patterns in order to control the acceleration associated with sitting back. Returning to the "lean forward" concept, many people bend their knees by first sinking their hips down and pushing their knees forward, in other words, they sit. This bends the knees but moves the hip back, or aft, of center, resulting in very little pressure on the tongue of their boots, and their hips aft of their feet.

The compensating body motion to counter this stance is shoulders-forward, however this makes you bend at the waist and puts the hips further back. The hip, the largest joint in the body, can create a lot of leverage in skiing; it can also create most of the problems if not positioned correctly.

When we break at the waist several things happen: First, we lose core strength in our midsection. Once the core is broken, there is strain on the lower back and too much strain on the thigh. Breaking at the waist, especially at the end of the turn, will create a stiff downhill leg. With a stiff leg, you will be unable to flex your ankle and knee. Most people brace or push the lower leg while bending at the waist to control speed, or brake at the end of the turn. This is not only inefficient but also exhausting, and usually results in a traverse between turns rather than a symmetrical transition, which puts the skier out of balance at the top of the next turn. On a steep slope this same stance will result in dipping the upper shoulder and dropping the uphill ski into the hill—which results in more instability.

So, what is the solution? Simple—stand up and move your hips over your feet during the transition of the turn. While reaching forward into the new pole plant with the downhill hand, shift your shoulder forward and down the hill, and tighten your core as you tip your skis into the new turn. This will load the tip of the ski and initiate the new turn with tip pressure. The result will be a carving ski with an even flow of snow from tip to tail. If done correctly, your skis will ease into the turn, and slightly accelerate at the end of the turn. And if you stand up and move your hips over your feet in the transition, you will remain in balance. Your ability to do this on varying terrain and conditions will allow you to expand your skiing experience.

We can't address pressure via hip and upper body alignment over the feet without talking about angulation, and herein lies the key to leaning forward—the stiffness of your ski boots. Boots are designed with varying degrees of stiffness, referred to as their "flex rating." Boots are constructed with a flex rating ranging from 60 to 140. On average, most boots fall within a 80 to 130 stiffness. The low end of the scale is a softer flexing boot, and the high end is a stiff or ridged flexing boot. Racers prefer stiffer boots.

Over the years, I have skied the entire range of boot flex. For a while, I was skiing in a 90-flex boot, which is considered soft by most advanced skiers' standards. But I enjoyed feeling my ankle flex to gain forward pressure and overall control. These days, I am back to skiing a 120 to 130 Dalbello boot flex, which I like mainly because the stiffer boot doesn't bottom out in moguls and aggressive moves on the steeps.

Here, again, we must address trends in skiing. These days, with the many shapes of skis, there are many flexing boots and no industry standard between brands, so a 130-flex in one brand could be 120 or less in another. This is due to plastic dynamics, and is better left to a designer to explain, however I do wish the industry would standardize this flex rating. The other varying part of boot design is cuff angle—the forward lean of a boot. The trend lately has been to straighten cuff angles, but in this case the knee is not over the toes.

I prefer boots with forward angle in the cuff. This places the knee over the toes and puts the ankle in a flexed position. There are varying reasons to use boots with a straight cuff, the biggest one being young skiers in parks, who prefer a straighter cuff for doing tricks and skiing backward. Hybrid boots that offer alpine touring options also have straighter cuffs because it is desirable for uphill travel. However, for performance alpine skiing where the intention is to make carving, powerful turns while remaining in balance, a boot with a forward-angled cuff provides the best performance.

Many of the skiers at my camps and clinics have boots that don't allow their knee to

9

move forward over their toes, and we must make them aware of this limitation and the affect it is having on their skiing.

Along with this line of thought, many parents are quick to put their young skiers in boots that are too stiff. Especially the racers. I would prefer that younger skiers understand and experience movement patterns that create a balanced ski stance rather than limit it, and traditional, stiff race boots limit movement patterns, which limits range of motion and overall balance.

Ok, so far we've explored hip placement and how it effects ski pressure, boot stiffness, and cuff angle. Now we can discuss creating angles, which enhances how we lean and move forward. This is the crux of getting forward motion. Because of the stiffness of boots, there is only so far the knee can actually move forward. With this limitation, how can we get further forward to create the tip pressure required for a turning ski? Simple—we create angles, starting with flexing the ankle and driving it to the inside of the turn. This is complemented by moving the hip forward while angling the knee into the hill. Then, move the hip into the turn while maintaining an upright upper body, with hands driving downhill.

The result of this form is forward pressure at the top of the turn. As we move through the turn the hips will sink low and the feet will move forward as the ski accelerates, then, by moving forward and standing up in the transition of the turn, you can realign your body over your feet in preparation for the next turn. The drills and skills outlined in this book, complemented by the videos in the ATS II App, will help you master the body motion needed for all-terrain skiing.

ALL-GRIP, NO-SLIP SKIING

ALL-GRIP, NO-SLIP SKIING IS AS much a state of mind as it is proper body positioning. Our skis' edges are designed to grip, cut, and hold onto the slope. They are sharp and should be used as a tool for fine-tuning your experience on the mountain.

At my clinic and camps at Big Sky, Montana, and in Europe as well, I encourage skiers to "Stand against the Mountain." What does this mean? Simply to lean out and away from the slope, which can be a bit scary at first. But remember, skis are designed for this. As you lean out and away from the slope, move your body toward the inside of the turn while allowing your skis to move out and away from your body. This will encourage proper body position, not only in the arc of the turn but also in the transition out of it. Your feet will naturally move under your hips, keeping you in balance and moving you forward toward the next turn.

Unfortunately, too many advanced skiers use their edges as a last-ditch effort to slow down, which causes the ski to skid and/or chatter. Skiers attending my clinics often report feeling their edges for the first time, thinking they'd done something wrong because the sensation was so different from their normal sliding ski turns.

Skiing requires us to be proactive in every movement, and the faster you go, the more you must anticipate your movements. You want to stand against the mountain because that edge grip provides the confidence to arc your skis on steep and firm conditions. A ski racer once told me, "Ski technique can be summed up this way: keep your body moving forward down the hill and fight to keep up with your skis."

Where does this leave the skier who does not want to ski as fast as a racer? The answer remains the same: move your body forward and over your feet for all-grip, no-slip skiing. Speed control is in the grip. The grip is in proper body position. The better the position, the better the grip. The better the grip, the more control you have.

Balance

BALANCE IS THE ISSUE FOR
ALL-TERRAIN SKIING

THE MORE I TEACH BACKCOUNTRY and big mountain skills to skiers, the more I realize that, for most advanced skiers, the problem is rarely a talent issue, rather, it's a balance issue. When it comes to turning a ski, the dynamics don't change much from groomed slopes to steep powdery pitches, but few skiers realize this. Fear and apprehension equal a lack of balance. For nearly two decades traditional ski schools have taught minimized motion when it comes to technique, and focused too much on tipping skis rather than turning skis. The common resulting issue for intermediate skiers comes when entering difficult terrain, such as trees, moguls, and steeps with no idea how to decelerate. This results in fear, which can throw you out of balance. Skiers can conquer apprehension and fear by practicing speed acceptance, slowly building confidence and successes when making challenging runs on new terrain.

Speed Acceptance. Skis are designed for acceleration, but deceleration happens over a series of turns. So, rather than skiing to slow down, practice skiing to accelerate. Decelerate in the last three turns of your descent. You can practice this on a groomed slope and gradually move to steeper terrain with cut-up snow or moguls.

Maximize Motion. When it comes to skiing powder, trees, and steeps, it's important to maximize motion. You can do this by reaching further down the hill with your pole plants, or standing taller between turns. When you maximize motion, you unlock your balance and are better able to control your speed.

You go where you look, so look where you want to go. The key to all-mountain skiing is looking down the hill past obstacles. Too often skiers tell me what they want to avoid, but rarely do they tell me where they want to turn. Focus your eyes beyond the mogul, tree, or rocks, and see the path around obstacles. Then decelerate over a series of two or three turns.

A balanced skier is a thing of beauty and, as skiers, our main job is to complement the terrain we ski. Breathe deeply, relax, and remember it's a balance issue, not a talent issue.

Balance is something we're all born with. It's instinctive and natural; we rarely think about it consciously. Basically, we were born to walk, run, skip, and jump. With this gift of balance comes trust—a subconscious trust of standing up and not falling over—whether we're walking, running, or participating in athletic activities. With this recognition of balance and trust in our natural abilities, we humans have been able to accomplish extraordinary athletic feats. Understanding the basics of balance is the key to understanding how to ski. I can't stress this enough. Ruedi Bear wrote, in his book *Ski Like the Best*, "When you ski, never get locked into any kind of firm position." Skiing is a dynamic sport. It is disastrous for your skiing to get stuck in a static position.

The following six drills are necessary to reacquaint you with your natural sense of balance on skis. They'll help you to trust in yourself and your instinctive abilities. Take the time to work your way through each lesson and perform all recommended sets of the exercises. Remember, each drill complements every other drill in the program. Build a strong foundation and practice, practice, practice.

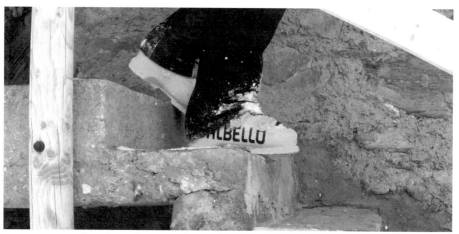

Step down the stairs placing the middle of the sole of your boot
on the outer edge of the stair.

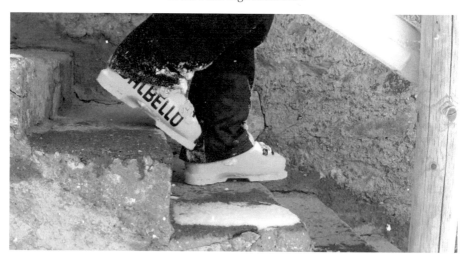

Roll the front of your boot down off the edge towards the next step.

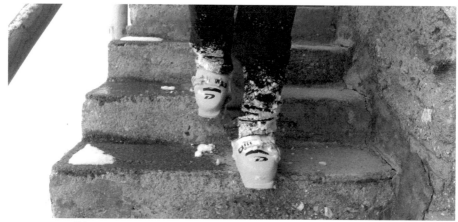

Place your opposite foot sole on the outer edge of the next step and
roll the toe of the boot towards the next step.

Balance

HOW TO WALK DOWN STAIRS IN SKI BOOTS

> **Goal:** To comfortably and safety walk down stairs in ski boots.
>
> **Body Position:** Place the center of the boot's sole on the edge of the stair, and roll your foot forward.
>
> Please refer to the ATS App for more instruction and the video demonstration of this drill.

SKI BOOTS ARE AWKWARD TO walk in. They are stiff, clunky, and their soles are often slippery—this can make walking down stairs scary. And because ski areas are located on mountains, there are always stairways to navigate in parking lots, lodges, and base areas.

So, what's the best way to walk down stairs in ski boots? The keys are where you step on the stair, and with what part of the boot.

When walking down stairs in ski boots, with one hand on the rail for balance, step down onto the stair below with the heel of your boot three to four inches back from the edge of the stair, so as you roll your foot forward, the center of the boot will land on the edge of the stair, with the front of the boot overhanging. This will allow your foot to smoothly roll forward and down the stair. Then, in a continuous motion, place your other foot on the stair below, striking the heel first with the center of the boot resting on the edge of the stair, and let that foot smoothly roll forward.

Practice this on a few stairs with no other people around, and with nothing in your hands. Remember to hold the rail with one hand and focus on being fluid, allowing your feet to flow and roll off each stair. As you gain confidence, increase the number of stairs you walk down without stopping. Try to keep your eyes up, not staring at your feet, this will give a great perspective of what is around you, and make you feel more comfortable.

The best practice for walking down stairs in a crowd while carrying your skis is to carry them in one hand, right above the bindings, placing the tails of the skis down on the stair beside the foot on the same side, both landing on the step at the same time. This adds stability, with one hand on the rail, one hand on the skis, and the tail of the skis helping you brace as you smoothly walk down. I always tuck the tip of the skis down toward my chest, so the tails point up, not back. Like all things, practice will help your confidence as you glide up and down stairs like a seasoned pro.

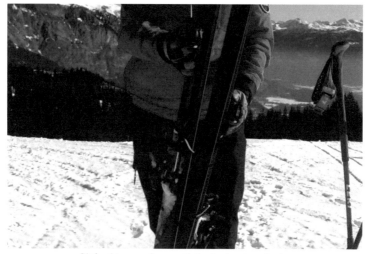

Slide skis together until the brakes interlock.

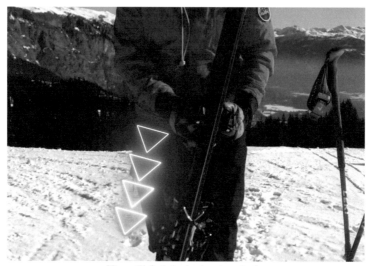

You will feel the brakes interlock

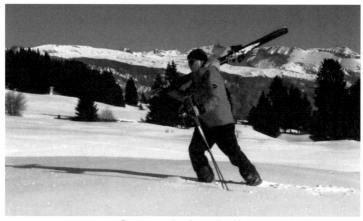

Go in search of powder :))

Balance

HOW TO CARRY YOUR SKIS

> **Goal:** To carry your skis without them sliding apart.
>
> **Body Position:** Skis on your shoulder, tips forward, with the brakes holding them together.
>
> Please refer to the ATS App for more instruction and the video demonstration of this drill.

SKIING REQUIRES LOTS OF EQUIPMENT and gear, and it seems there's no end in sight for new gadgets—earphones for music, boot and hand warmers, and apps that talk to us while we ski. Every year we stuff more items inside our backpack or boot bag to go ski. It makes me laugh, how we can complicate the simple pleasure of skiing.

I like the basics of the sport: people, mountains, snow, skis, boots, bindings, hat, gloves, and warm clothing are really all that is required. Over the years, as I've witnessed the growth in popularity of gadgets, I've also seen firsthand the decline of the simpler skills, like how to carry your skis.

One winter, while filming in St. Anton, our guide Jans, a Dutch national who'd married into a local family, was hiking us up a ridge to drop down a big face of powder slope on the St. Christoph side of the resort. It was a short, steep hike, and he encouraged us to throw our skis over our shoulder and scurry up the ridge. What impressed me about his guiding technique was his attention to detail through every phase of being on the mountain. Hiking with our skis over our shoulders was no different.

He did a simple demonstration on how to make sure your skis won't slip apart while hiking. It wasn't brain surgery, and most of our group was seasoned professionals, but nevertheless he took the few minutes to review the proven technique.

He took one ski, faced the base away from him, then took the other ski, lifted it up, and slid it down onto the first ski so the brakes locked, then picked up both skis with the first ski, allowing the brakes to lift the second ski.

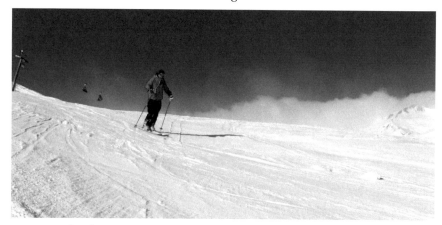

Leading with your chest, ski straight downhill on flat parallel skis.
Stay perpendicular to the slope Keep head up, eyes forward

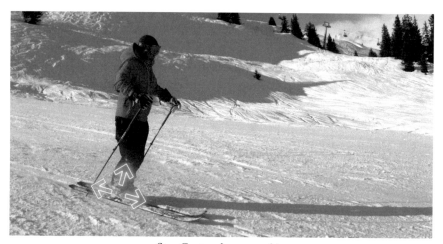

Stay Centered on your skis

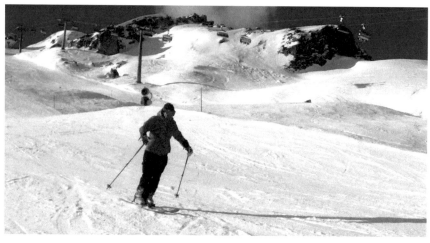

Lean Forward and feel the acceleration

Balance

GRAVITY PULL

●

Goal: To experience the pull of gravity and the glide of a flat ski.
Body Position: Ski straight downhill, body perpendicular to the slope
Please refer to the ATS App for more instruction and
the video demonstration of this drill.

IN HER BOOK, *THE CENTERED SKIER,* Denise McCluggage says: "What is an essential difference between a good skier and a poor skier? It is their relationship with the mountain." To form that relationship, we must understand gravity's effect on our bodies.

Most beginners have trouble because they haven't yet established a relationship with gravity. Too many factors can change at once. You're on a steep mountain slope, you're in the snow, and you're wearing skis and big clodhopper boots.

In mastering this drill, you'll learn efficient use of your body in relation to gravity. Simply put, you'll learn how gravity pulls your body down the fall line, which will enhance your mobility and fluidity. Remember, skiing is about constant fluidity; any kind of rigidity is a no-no.

You must learn to keep your body erect and perpendicular to the slope. Internalize how easily your feet move when gravity is pulling you from the center of your chest. This weightlessness on your feet will make it much easier to turn your skis.

We're going to practice the Gravity Pull to experience gravity in action. On a gentle slope, face downhill in a snowplow stop. Now, start to ski straight down the hill, leading with your chest—this will keep you perpendicular to the slope. Be sure to keep your head up and your eyes looking forward.

As you start to move, you'll immediately experience acceleration combined with a feeling of weightlessness, as if you're gliding through air, and you will clearly feel slight acceleration. This is due to the way you're holding your body, allowing gravity to pull your body forward from your chest while keeping yourself erect and centered. Gravity does all the work for you. You'll exert minimal effort and get maximum efficiency in return. Go twenty to thirty feet, then stop.

This drill is a great way to learn how the flat ski feels and performs when your body is perpendicular to the slope—the natural way to accelerate. It also shows you how to conserve energy and increase efficiency. I often find it's the best way—especially when I'm tired—to let gravity and balance get me down the hill.

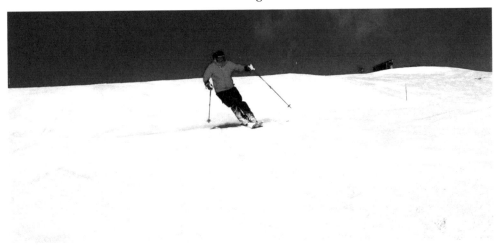

Stand tall in your Gravity Pull Stance, start to ski and
create angles with no compression

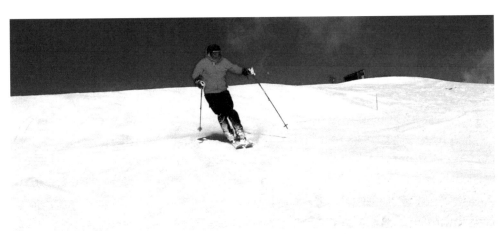

Allow your skis to float under you as you move to the next turn

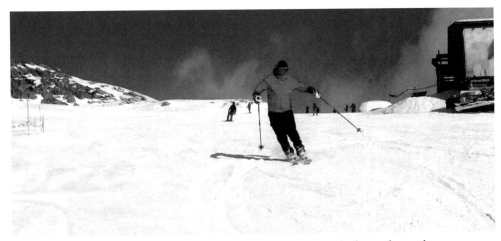

Experience how effortless it is to ski by shifting your weight from side to side.

FLOATING TURNS

> **Goal:** To experience how proper body position can turn a ski without using strength.
>
> **Body Position:** Standing tall on your skis, glide down the slope creating angles
>
> Please refer to the ATS App for more instruction and
> the video demonstration of this drill.

SKIING WELL IS ABOUT POSITION, not strength. When a skier is in the proper position, turning takes less energy. In the Gravity Pull drill we experienced how, when we stand tall with our hips forward, gravity does the work. Now we'll talk about turning in an efficient manner, without relying on our strength.

This is a good time to contemplate one of my favorite riddles: Do we turn the skis or do the skis turn us? Although there may not be a simple, clear answer that satisfies every situation, for the purpose of this drill we want to experience the ski turning us, not the skier turning the ski.

The ski is designed to turn, and this drill will help you feel how, when in the right position, the ski will turn itself. As I've pointed out, because of new shapes and designs in skis, many skiers control their speed by dropping their hips and twisting their feet. This technique is not only inefficient, it also requires a lot of strength, which eventually causes fatigue.

The Floating Turns drill is designed to illustrate the importance of gravity and angulation. On a gentle, groomed slope, stand tall, like you did in Gravity Pull, and point your skis straight down the slope as you push off and gain a little speed, slowly moving your hips in the direction you want to go, feeling the skis move in that direction. Then, slowly move your hips over and across the skis in the opposite direction, feeling the skis drift in that direction. Making long, slow turns, resist dropping your hips, twisting your feet, or making sharp turns.

Make four to six turns, then stop, regroup, and do it again. This exercise should feel effortless, and your skis should float under your body. The more angle you create, the more the ski is tipped, and the more the edges grip the snow.

Observe your skiing form, and adjust as needed. If you feel your hips sinking down, stand taller. If you are twisting your feet, be patient and allow the ski to dictate the radius of the turn instead.

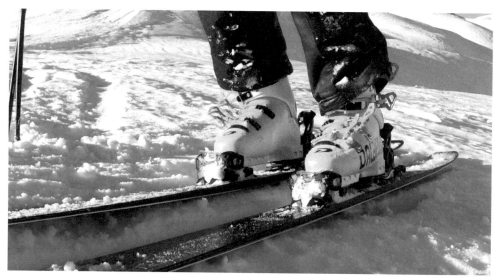

Lift the buckles of your boots

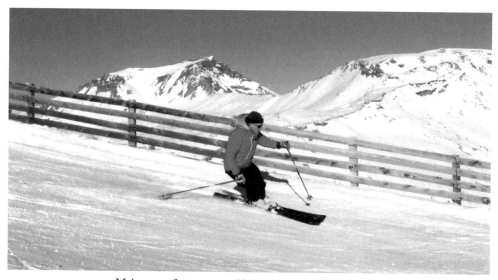

Make turns flexing you ankles and feeling your boots flex

Balance

LOOSE BOOTS

■

> **Goal:** To identify your center without relying on your boots.
>
> **Body Position:** Make large radius turns with boots unbuckled; rock back and forth between your heels and toes.
>
> Please refer to the ATS App for more instruction and the video demonstration of this drill.

IN SKIING, BALANCE IS WHAT everyone must master in order to reach new levels of ability. The best drill for discovering natural balance is skiing with Loose Boots. You can begin practicing this drill in your living room before you head out to the slope. Slip into your boots and latch the buckles loosely. Now stand in skiing position and push your knees forward. You should feel your shins press into the boot tongue while rocking between your toes and heels. Move your body from the hips down as if you were skiing, and give your boots a real workout as you flex them. You'll feel your feet—not your boots—as they move.

Now you're ready to try this on the slopes. Snap into your bindings with your boots still loosely buckled, and begin skiing. Take a couple of runs on a slope that is below your ability level, making easy, medium radius turns. Go slowly—you may feel slightly out of control at first, as it makes turning difficult. Start off with wide, sweeping giant slalom turns until your confidence grows. Next, start to ski more down the fall line, making sharper, shorter turns.

No longer relying on the safeguard and support of your boots, instinct will adjust your skiing stance accordingly and ensure your body remains balanced. Remain flexible and adapt your body to the changing terrain. Stay forward in your boots by curling your toes. That one little action will bring your whole body forward and allow you to stand up strong, balanced, and in the center of your skis. The old saying, "keep on your toes," applies to every sport.

Arms and hands play a huge part in the balanced ski stance. Keep upper body movement limited. Here's a good tip to remember: if you can't see both arms, then they are out of position. Don't confuse a quiet, strong upper body with a stiff and tense upper body. The biggest benefits in raising your skill level come when you are relaxed and fluid, calm and strong. Your comfort level will grow after a couple of runs. Often, I forget that my boots are loose! When that happens, progress is being made. Subconsciously, I'm adjusting my stance on my skis and trusting my natural instincts. When you reach this point, take on more challenging terrain. Progress slowly and continue making wide, sweeping giant slalom turns. Once you feel confident, start to ski more in the fall line with shorter radius turns.

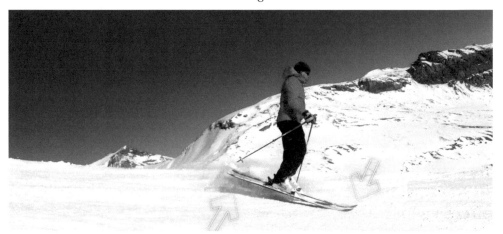

Start to ski and jump up pulling your heels up while leaving your tips on the snow

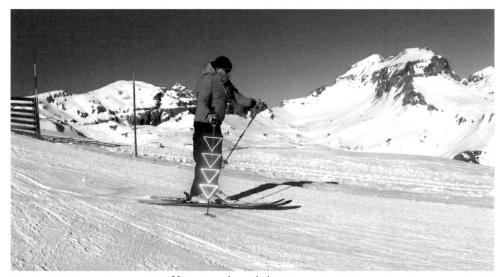

Use your poles to help you pop up

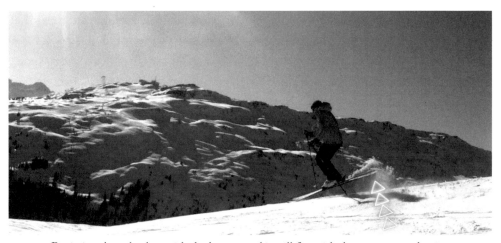

By timing the pole plant with the hop, your skis will flex with the pressure on the tips

Balance

TIP HOPS

> **Goal:** To introduce the concept of retraction.
>
> **Body Position:** Make small hop-turns, keeping ski tips on the snow and lifting the tails up and off the snow.
>
> Please refer to the ATS App for more instruction and the video demonstration of this drill.

DYNAMIC MOTION IS A BIG part of skiing. This drill, Tip Hops, will be the foundation for much of the motion required for all-terrain skiing. One of the main reasons it is important to have your hips over your feet is so you can be in an athletic stance and gain mobility—this drill will introduce you to dynamic motion. The concept of retraction is a major part of all-terrain skiing—mogul skiers use it, big mountain skiers use it in all sorts of conditions, and when it comes to steep skiing it is far more efficient to pull your feet up and under your hips than it is to drop your hips down and aft of your feet.

To start with, stand on a flat surface with your skis on and simply jump up, keeping your ski tips on the snow. Make small hops, pulling your heels up toward your hips. The key here is to pull the tails of your skis up higher than their tips. Use your poles for stability and leverage. You can brace against them to help you get up off the snow. Don't make a large jump, this is a hop, just pull your heels up under your hips.

Once you can do this consistently, you're ready to do it while skiing. This drill is best done on an intermediate slope with a bit more angle then the drills we've practiced thus far. Begin skiing down the hill, making three small hops without turning, focusing on the tails of your skis coming up off the snow. If you can do three or four sets of hops in a straight line, you're ready to add a turn.

Once you get a bit of momentum, make a pole plant, as you do, hop up slightly, pulling your heels up and under your hips while keeping the tips of your skis on the snow. As you do this, pivot your feet out to the side and land in a turn. The key here is to keep the momentum, and just after your feet are back on the snow, initiate another hop by planting the other pole and repeating the motion for the next turn.

This drill takes timing and coordination, so be easy on yourself as you explore this movement. The timing of the pole plant is a major part of the coordination of this drill. Stand up, move forward, and start moving down the hill. If you're struggling with this drill, leave it and come back to it another time. This is an advanced drill and, as you progress through this program, it will become easier.

PLANT YOUR POLE IN GRAVITY

THE FOCUS IN ALL-TERRAIN SKIING is on keeping your motion going in the direction of gravity. Pole-planting initiates the skier's motion down the hill. Problems occur when pole plants are angled in the direction of the ski tips, or across the hill. Your poles should always be planted at right angles to your feet.

Ultimately, you want the tip of the pole point in the direction of your path. When the pole's tip travels down the fall line, several things happen: your shoulder creates a counter-angle to your skis, your hips move toward your hands, your skis release in the fall line, and your eyes look down the fall line.

At my camps around the world, we dig a bit deeper into this concept and explore these four points:

When you reach downhill with your pole plant, your shoulders do two things: they square off to the fall line, and move out and over your feet. This gives you more speed control.

Now you are ready for the transition of the turn. If you move your hips and core toward your downhill pole in the fall line, you'll move your body out and over your feet. This sets you up for a smoother transition.

What you discover in these movements is how the skis seem to release and flow into the fall line, traveling out and away from your body. This sets you up for a smooth, round turn with your upper body moving through the center of the arc. The result is more control and less energy expenditure.

The bonus is, when you plant your pole in the direction of the fall line, your eyes are looking down the hill rather than across it. This points you into the flow, and you'll make turns with greater confidence.

So, planting your pole in gravity, or down the fall line, will set up a chain reaction that makes you more efficient, expends less energy, and makes skiing more dynamic.

The key is resisting the temptation to swing the tip of the pole in the direction of the tip of the ski. Doing so moves your body across the hill rather than down it, so your body moves *around* the arc rather than powering *through* it. Plus, once your eyes are focused down the hill, you'll be less intimidated by obstacles in your path. In the Upper Body chapter, I'll address pole planting—how it enhances our balance and keeps us in the fall line.

The drills in this chapter will help you achieve the goal of having a calm and strong upper body. Look Down the Hill teaches you to see beyond any perceived obstacles. Pole Clapping will teach you to "keep 'em where you can see 'em." Poles Behind Your Back will make you aware of upper body rotation. Ski Without Poles, I believe, is the most liberating drill in this program. Pole Point and Mogul Pole are the two most important pole planting drills. Downhill Hand Sweep illustrates the importance of the skier's upper body and its relationship to the lower body. Remember, economical movement equals less energy wasted. These drills will help make you more efficient, and get you skiing at your maximum potential.

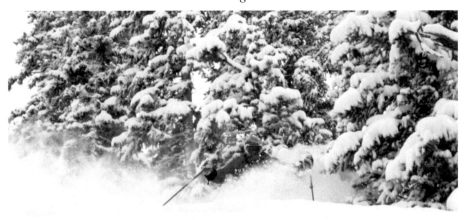

Point your head downhill and your eyes down the fall line.

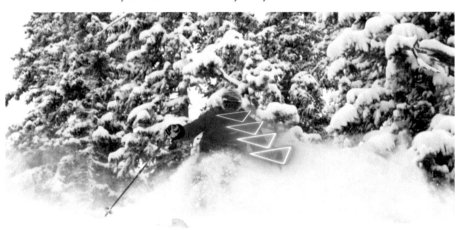

This will keep your shoulders square to the hill.

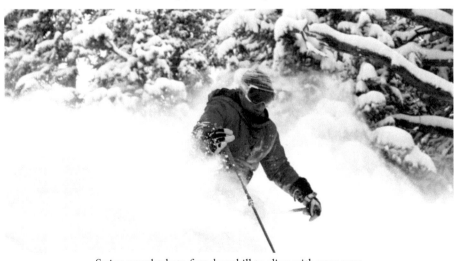

Swing your body to face downhill to align with your eyes.

LOOK DOWN THE HILL

●

> **Goal:** To demonstrate how your body goes where you look.
> **Body Position:** Ski with your head up and eyes looking down the fall line.
> Please refer to the ATS App for more instruction and
> the video demonstration of this drill.

IT IS IMPORTANT TO MAXIMIZE the relationship between yourself and the mountain. Skiers of all abilities can't afford to be startled by obstacles or changes in terrain. Our eyes prepare our other senses for what lies ahead. Learning how to better use our vision helps overcome a natural fear of steeper slopes, changing snow conditions, and obstacles.

Look Down the Hill teaches proper body positioning. Your shoulders are straight, arms out in front of your body, and head positioned so you're looking down the hill. Don't let the simplicity of this drill fool you. Looking down the hill has many benefits—for instance, your body will go where you look. If you're looking off to the side, you aren't skiing downhill. Big mountain ski legend Dean Decas says, "The biggest improvement I see in skiers is when they learn to look down the hill past obstacles that used to cause them fear or disrupt their focus."

Start this drill on any slope you're comfortable with, and face downhill. Begin skiing, making sure your head is pointing downhill and your eyes are looking straight down the fall line. Your head is the key to athletic motion; looking ahead will square your shoulders to the hill. This is the best position for your body. Dan's ATS II App and accompanying images show the skier's eyes looking down the hill as their body moves into the best skiing position.

Now begin to traverse. Let your skis run across the hill, keeping your head up and eyes looking down the fall line. As you begin to make your turn, swing your body to face downhill and align with your eyes. Continue looking down the fall line as you begin to traverse in the opposite direction. Feel how your eyes guide you.

The interesting thing about following your gaze is how you'll instinctively keep to the fall line and intuitively ski the path of least resistance. This enhances your relationship with the mountain and smooths out your skiing style without any major adjustments in skiing technique. Once again, it is proven that when our body is in the right position, skiing becomes easier.

Now you have a new tool for overcoming the fears of striking an obstacle or unexpected changes in snow conditions. Just look past it, to where you want to go—which is downhill. This active visualization will focus your eyes down the hill, and you'll ski exactly where you want to go.

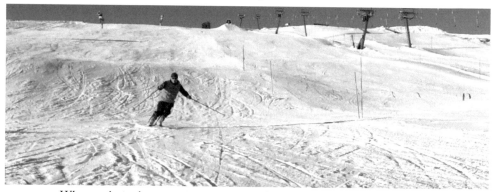

When you're in the turn, raise your arms in front and prepare to cross your poles.

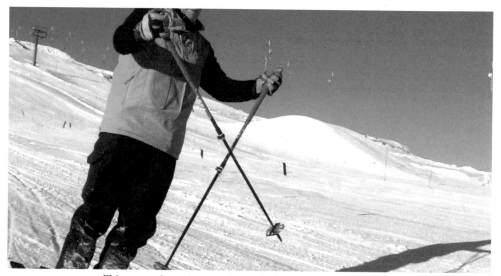

Take note of your hand position while your poles are in the X.

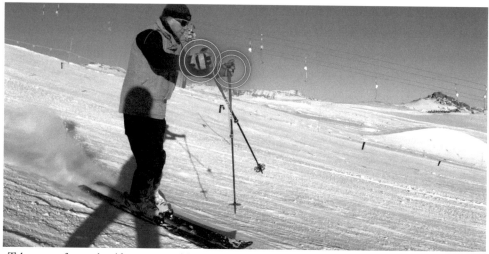

Take note of your shoulders position. They are square with the hill, your body is pointed down the fall line. Where they should be.

POLE CLAPPING

> **Goal:** To develop constant, fluid motion, and isolation and separation of certain body parts.
>
> **Body Position:** Ski, clicking your poles instead of doing pole plants.
>
> Please refer to the ATS App for more instruction and
> the video demonstration of this drill.

I CALL SKI POLES "TWIZZLE Sticks" because many skiers don't understand how to correctly utilize them. As a result, misuse of poles can impede a relaxed, fluid style of skiing. Pole Clapping is a drill to improve your use of poles. As you practice, you will learn more about the isolation and separation of body parts. You'll find out where your hands and arms are—and where they're supposed to be. You will also learn the importance of hand position in relation to your overall balance. Begin skiing down any slope you're comfortable with. Once you're moving, start making short radius turns. When you're in the turn, raise your arms in front and cross your poles, clicking them together. As you make the X with your poles, look at the position of your hands—the illustration in Dan's ATS II App clearly shows this natural hand position—they're out in front of your body, exactly where they should be, while your head and eyes are pointed downhill.

Next time you cross and clap, notice the position of your shoulders. They are square with the hill and your body is pointed directly downhill, on the fall line. Once again, this is exactly where everything should be. Continue your pole claps, noticing how the motion of clicking the poles and making the X is in your wrists. Similarly, whenever you make a pole plant, the motion should only be in your wrist.

This is what I mean by the separation and isolation of body parts. Once you see and feel where the individual parts are, reintegrate them into your whole-body sense. Combine what you're doing in the drill with a smooth, fluid motion. Put it all together and feel yourself skiing better. This drill takes the focus off skiing technique and places it on your natural ability. Internalize the isolation and separation of your whole body from your feet, knees, and hips, right through to your head, shoulders, and hands.

Create your own clapping rhythm while you ski—this will help you gain confidence. More importantly, it shows how you can make quicker, gentler pole plants. You don't need to stab at the snow. A light touch is much more efficient, and minimizes effort and movement.

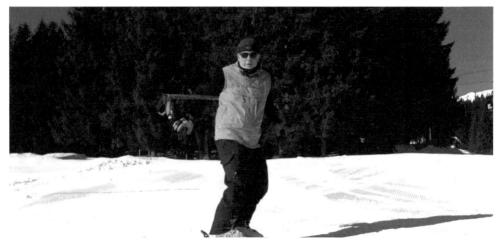

Take both poles in one hand and swing them around your back. Fold your elbows around them to hold them across the middle of your back.

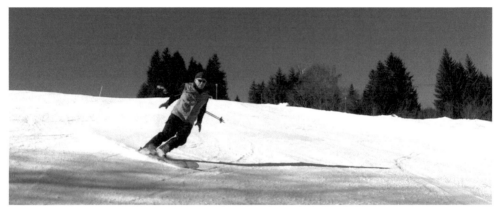

Now, square your shoulders down the hill and ski.

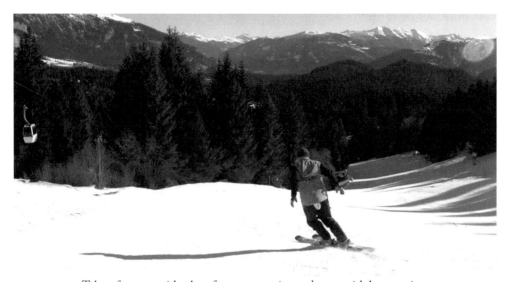

Take a few runs with a lot of counter rotation and some with less rotation.

POLES BEHIND YOUR BACK

Goal: To develop a calm, strong upper body while illustrating isolation and separation of the upper and lower body.

Body Position: Ski an intermediate run with both poles behind your back, elbows folded around them.

Please refer to the ATS App for more instruction and the video demonstration of this drill.

SKIING WITH YOUR POLES BEHIND your back is the fastest way to diagnose whether you have too much upper body rotation. This drill will also help you understand how counter-rotation with your upper body can and will increase overall stability on an angled edge. Ultimately, as you ski and adjust your upper body rotation while simultaneously adjusting hip and knee angulation, you will experience and fine-tune your overall body movements.

Skiing on a well-groomed intermediate trail, take both poles in one hand, swing them around your back, and hold them across the middle of your back by folding your elbows around them. Make six to eight medium to large radius turns, using as much of the slope as you like, then stop, regroup, and do it again.

Your first few tries will probably feel restricted and awkward. With this drill, there is a tendency to bend at the waist—remind yourself to stand tall, and don't break at the waist. Once you start feeling comfortable, observe what is happening with your upper body position in the turns, and in the transitions between them. Don't attempt to make any major changes, just observe what direction your shoulders are facing. On your third and fourth runs skiing with your poles behind your back, start to experiment with shoulder position. Start by squaring them down the hill, and ski a few sections of trail that way. Then ski a few sections with slightly less counter-rotation, splitting the difference between having your shoulders face the direction of your ski and completely square to the hill. Somewhere between these two positions, you will start to feel comfortable and stable.

Then try a few runs with a lot of counter-rotation. Try going past square, really stretching the upper body to face down the hill. Practice this for a few runs, increasing the number of turns you're making, and just free ski with your poles behind your back. Make adjustments that feel good and enhance your performance. After a few runs, your natural position will start to reveal itself.

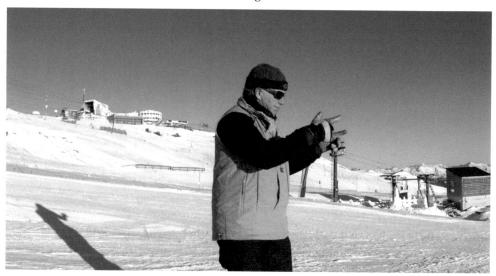

This drill is fun and helps you to discover the freedom of skiing.

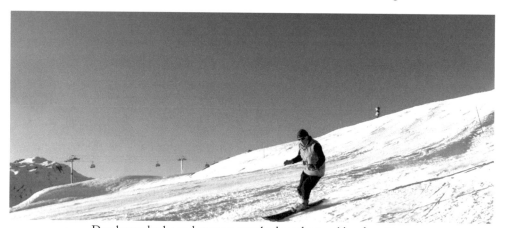

Develop and calm and strong upper body and natural hand position.

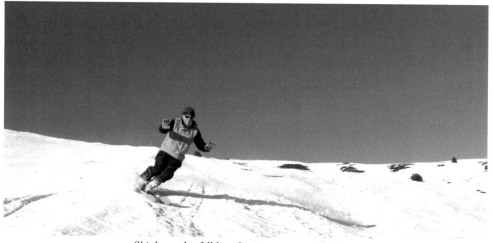

Ski down the fall line, letting your arms be free.

SKI WITHOUT POLES

●

> **Goal:** To develop a calm, strong upper body and natural hand position while skiing.
>
> **Body Position:** Ski without poles on any run you are comfortable with.
>
> Please refer to the ATS App for more instruction and the video demonstration of this drill.

TO DISCOVER JOY, CONFIDENCE, AND natural body position while skiing, I find taking away a skier's poles is the most direct way to obtain these goals. Plus, it's fun to see their face at the top of a lift when I quietly collect their poles and lean them up against a ski rack or under a tree. Unannounced and without much fanfare, the realization that we're about to head off down a glade run, mogul field, or steep pitch without the aid of ski poles gets their attention real quick.

I just turn and say, "Follow me!" and head off down the trail. Once people are over the initial shock, you can start to see the transformation in their body stance. In general, when talking to a group without poles, I'll reference how the upper body dictates lower body performance, and how the hands naturally find their proper position out in front and down the hill. Then we start skiing longer sections of trail, slowly skiing more challenging terrain, and the results are amazing. Skiers start to find their flow and, in a few runs, seem to totally forget all about their poles at the top of the mountain, several lift rides away.

The freedom found in skiing without poles is almost instant because we are balanced creatures and, often, finding our balance point is easier than we make it out to be. This drill is effective for all abilities and terrain. Once hands are freed from carrying poles, we don't have to think about the timing of pole plants, where to hold our hands, and so forth. Give this a try once every ski trip, and be amazed at the results.

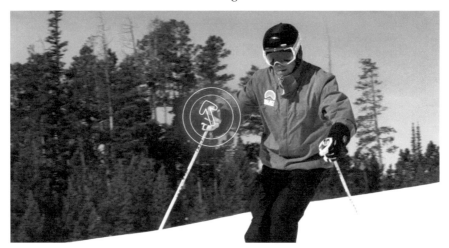

As you start to ski, cock one wrist so your index finger points up and your pole tip extends forward.

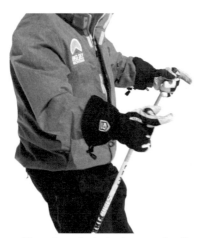

Plant the pole tip in the snow, leveling your index finger to point forward again.

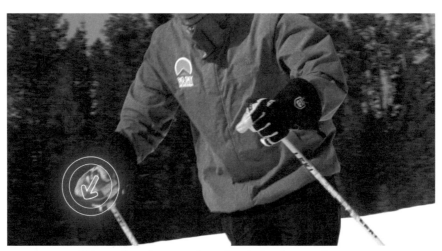

Ski past the pole so your finger is pointing down at the snow

POLE POINT

> **Goal:** To develop a proper pole plant and hand position.
> **Body Position:** Hold your poles with both index fingers pointing down the fall line.
>
> Please refer to the ATS App for more instruction and
> the video demonstration of this drill.

NOW THAT YOU'VE SKIED WITHOUT poles, practicing proper hand, arm, and upper body position, you're ready to learn how to use your poles properly. The Pole Point drill will combine what you've learned in all the previous Upper Body drills.

Get yourself on a comfortable slope with your hands holding your poles out in front of your body in a relaxed position. Now, point your index fingers downhill, right at the place where you're looking. Keep your head up, shoulders square to the hill.

Begin skiing the fall line. As you move forward, extend the tip of one pole by cocking your wrist so your index finger points up. Plant the tip of the pole in the snow. As you do, your index finger will level out. Ski past the planted pole, so your index finger is pointing down at the snow. As you turn, repeat the motion with the other pole. Don't swing your whole upper body or stab at the snow. The important motion is in the snap of the wrist. Keep your index fingers pointed to give you a reference for the proper motion. As demonstrated in Dan's ATS II App, develop a smooth, easy motion using your wrists, not your shoulders. Plant one pole tip, moving your arm forward to the extent of your reach. Point the opposite pole tip out in front of your body, and repeat the motion. Chant this mantra: *Point, plant, push.* Continue this smooth, rhythmic motion until you have a natural feeling of wrist movement. Notice how your shoulders stay square to the hill and do not rotate. Notice how your arms stay bent in a relaxed way, moving forward and backward as your poles and index fingers point the way down the hill.

Practice this motion on or off the snow. Mastering this drill will allow you to use your poles instinctively. Pole Point further emphasizes the isolation and separation of body parts, in this case the arms and wrists. Notice how, because of the previous drills where you did not use your poles, they have now become a natural extension of your body. Also note that, when you didn't use your poles, in Ski Without Poles, you naturally held your hands out in front of your body. This drill also reminds you to always keep your hands out in front, where you can see and use them.

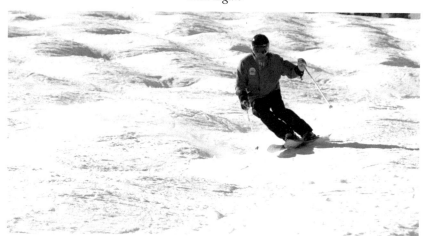

Grasp the poles gently and point your index fingers down the fall line.

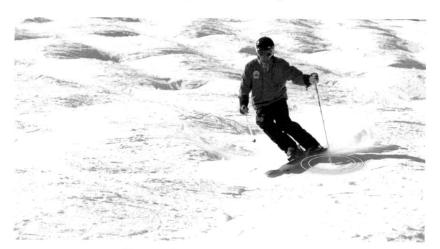

Focus on the pole plant and not turning.

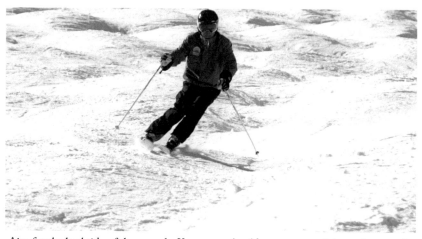

Aim for the backside of the moguls. Keep your shoulders square, anticipate the moguls, reach downhill and keep your body perpendicular to the hill.

MOGUL POLE

■

> **Goal:** To develop quick pole plants in moguls.
>
> **Body Position:** Practice rhythmic pole plants through a mogul field, aiming for the back sides of the moguls.
>
> Please refer to the ATS App for more instruction and the video demonstration of this drill.

THIS EXERCISE ELEVATES THE UPPER Body drills to a new level as you begin skiing more challenging terrain: the mogul fields. Now you're going to see how effective pole pointing can be. Mogul skiing depends on a quiet upper body. Check Dan's ATS II App to see the skiers' legs pumping like pistons while their upper bodies remain calm, upright, and facing straight down the fall line. Mogul Pole teaches how to use your poles to maintain upper body poise while your feet and skis fly over and around moguls. Quick, precise pole plants are essential to successful mogul skiing. Begin by skiing a small mogul field that is not too steep. Face your upper body downhill, holding your arms out in front. Grasp the poles gently and point your index fingers down the fall line. The goal here is to focus on pole plants and not worry about turning.

Plant a pole and use the same movement you learned in Pole Point: *point, plant, push.* Move your wrist forward as you aim for the back side of the mogul. Keep your hands visible. Always try to plant the tip of your pole on the back side of the mogul. If you plant on the front side, your pole will get jammed; as you ski past it, your arm will be forced out to the side, beyond your body, and will probably cause you to lose control.

Planting on the back side has many benefits: it allows natural hand and arm movement, keeps your shoulders square to the hill, allows you to better anticipate the mogul, and forces you to reach down the hill, which keeps your body perpendicular to the hill. You want to leverage your body up and over the mogul. Ski from the back to the front of the mogul, always maintaining a continuous, dynamic motion. Chant the mantra: *point, plant, push; point, plant, push.*

Notice on Dan's ATS II App how smoothly and quickly the skier moves from bump to bump. Remember to point your index finger to drive home the goal of this drill. Slow down and concentrate on your pole plants. Continue this drill until you feel confident on the small mogul field, then increase the intensity, either on more challenging terrain or by increasing your speed. Ski like the pros. Concentrate on your hands and your feet will follow. You'll see your skiing skills improve dramatically!

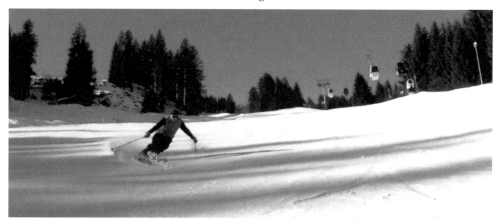

Sweeping your hand past your boot through the turn.

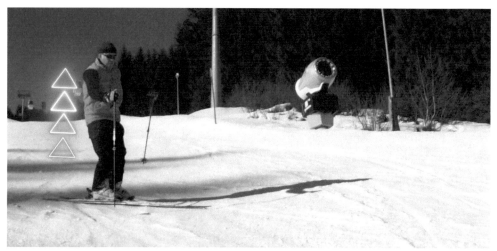

Remember to keep your upper body straight, shoulders square to the hill, and eyes looking downhill in the transition of the turn.

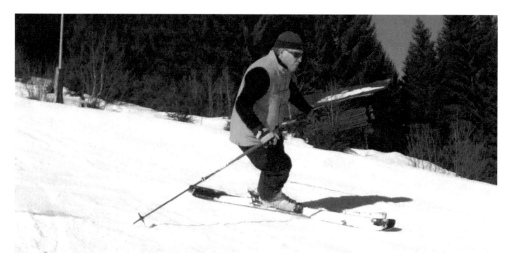

In the new turn reach for your boot again and sweep your hand back to the original position.

DOWNHILL HAND SWEEP

> **Goal:** To illustrate how proper positioning of the upper body will completely control the lower body.
>
> **Body Position:** While skiing large radius turns, sweep your downhill hand past your boot.
>
> Please refer to the ATS App for more instruction and the video demonstration of this drill.

MANY SKIERS, NOT KNOWING BETTER, ski with their feet and legs. No wonder they're exhausted by lunchtime! What they don't realize is this: the upper body rules! The lower body always follows the upper body. Your upper body helps you to balance, provides power, sustains fluid motion, and controls agility. The movements you'll make here will amaze you—almost like doing yoga while you're skiing! We're going to exaggerate upper body movement to display its power over the lower body. By the time you finish this drill, you'll understand how proper body mechanics are more important than ski technique.

Mastering this exercise helps you forget about foot steering, ankle pressure, and all the other terms that clog the mind. Focus instead on your body movement. Start skiing down a wide slope where you can make big, easy turns. Begin a traverse, raising your arms near shoulder level. Now, concentrate only on your arms as you move your uphill shoulder around. You'll feel yourself beginning to turn. Reach downhill with your hand as if you were going to touch your boot. At the same time, reach up into the air with your other hand, in the same direction.

Continue sweeping your hand past your boot, through the turn, and back up into the original position. At the same time, continue by bringing your new uphill hand into the downhill sweep, reversing the direction of your turn. Reach for your boot again, and sweep your hand back up to the original position. The sweeping motion creates momentum, while the bending motion forces you to flex your knees and push pressure down on your boots and skis. Sweeping your hand past your downhill boot—and back to the original position—unweights your skis and allows you to finish your turn with the tail of your skis. The result is a smooth, round turn with dynamic body movement, keeping you in an athletic, mobile stance while in constant motion.

As you perform one Downhill Hand Sweep after another, you'll begin to feel the gracefulness of making smooth, rounded turns. This is the capstone exercise for upper body positioning, essential to your success as an all-terrain skier.

Power

SKIING IN THE POWER POSITION

NOW THAT YOU KNOW ABOUT Balance and the importance of the Upper Body, you are ready to add Power to your stance and skiing positions. You'll focus first on the elements of a powerful stance in the Power Position and Power Position Turn drills. Then you'll begin focusing on the ski.

The Power drills are designed to help you master the three Foundational Skills: sliding, edging, and carving. The Foundational Skills begin with understanding your body and its positions, which in turn helps you achieve control of your skis. Remember not to spend too much time on any one drill. Remain fresh and alert by taking breaks, free skiing to give your body a chance to practice what it learned.

It is important to understand the Power Position before putting it in motion and attempting to integrate it into your skiing. Many skiers enter what I call the Frozen Zone at some point in a turn. This happens when the body loses its mobility from being out of balance. Out of balance means out of alignment. Skiers need to constantly check alignment in order to stay balanced and avoid injury or accidents.

Good skiers are in constant motion; they never remain in any one position. For example, watch a pro mogul event or downhill ski race. Notice that the skiers are always moving, up and down or side to side. These pro skiers are in fluid motion, constantly adjusting their balance to the ever-changing terrain. They are skiing from the Power Position. Finding your Power Position will give you more control and confidence, freeing you from the Frozen Zone and giving you the freedom to be dynamic and adaptable.

It has been said that the essence of skiing is in the turn—in the time and space when your body experiences a mix of forces: centrifugal force, gravity, friction, and acceleration. This elemental power is sometimes fluid and graceful, and at other times explosive and dynamic. The power in skiing is hidden within the skier. Each of us shapes our own outcome and leaves behind only a path through the snow.

Many skiers finish a well-groomed Blue Square or demanding Black Diamond feeling exhilarated and filled with the power of skiing. Hours later, driving home, we still feel this power and carry it back into our daily life as a sustaining force of empowerment. The best explanation I've heard is that this elemental power is the feeling of being alive. When I put my skis on, I'm a different person. I feel an unexplainable joy and happiness. After so many years of skiing, I still love it. It gives me a confident feeling about myself that stays with me in everything I do.

The Power Slide drill teaches the importance of a flat ski and what it feels like to slide a ski. The Power Slide to Traverse teaches the difference between a sliding and an edged ski. Power Slide to Carve illustrates the difference between edging and carving. Slowing and Flowing Turns and the Long Turns for Stability are two drills that combine all the teachings in this book. Mastering these two drills will build your confidence to a new level. Learning the techniques in this chapter will prepare you to enter the Zone of Excellence.

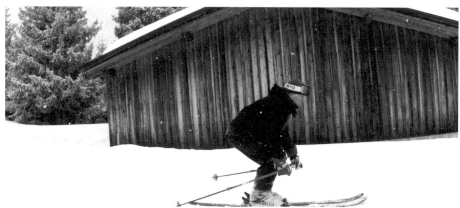

Crouch down. Then, jump straight into the air without using your poles

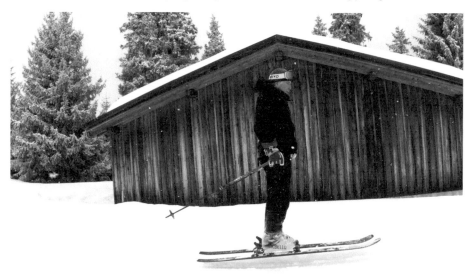

Make sure your skis remain parallel as they clear the ground.

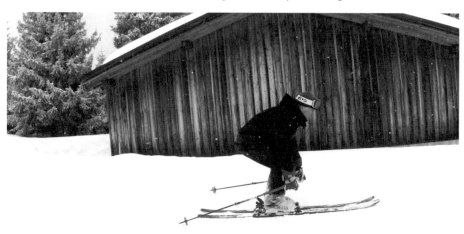

As you land, compress. Bend at the knees, and bring your upper body all the way down, as far as you can

Power

POWER POSITION

> **Goal:** To define your Power Position as an athletic stance in constant fluid motion.
>
> **Body Position:** Stand in an athletic position on a flat surface with skis on. Jump up and down three times. Then do the jumps while in motion.
>
> Please refer to the ATS App for more instruction and the video demonstration of this drill.

THE POWER POSITION DRILL IDENTIFIES how power is generated in skiing. The most important point of this lesson is that the Power Position changes throughout the turn. Therefore, skiers must sustain a mobile, athletic stance throughout every phase of the turn.

This drill sets the tone for all the Power drills. Balanced skiers with quiet upper bodies are on their way to becoming powerful skiers. While practicing this drill, concentrate on feeling the flow of your movements. Be relaxed, yet also dynamic and explosive. The Power Position helps you develop an athletic stance while in constant fluid motion.

You won't even need a slope to perform this drill. Instead, find a flat area and stand with your skis shoulder-width apart and your hands out in front, holding your ski poles. Crouch down, then jump straight into the air without using your poles. Make sure your skis clear the ground, keeping them parallel to each other and perpendicular to the ground, aiming to be balanced and smooth. Try not to let them slap down upon landing. The secret is in moving from the body's center. Use the ball of the foot to take off and land on; absorb with the legs. Limit arm movement and be certain not to bend at the waist. When you land, let your entire body compress. Bend your knees and bring your upper body all the way down, as far as you can. Absorb the entire landing and jump again—do three jumps.

The Power Position occurs between the first and second jump. From the time you land to the time you take off, the body is mobile, balanced, and in a constant state of motion. When the body is balanced and mobile, it can adjust to changes in terrain, speed, and position.

In fact, the whole range of movement is intrinsic to the Power Position. Why? Because no single stage of the jump can exist without the prior stage.

Power drives the whole act; Position is our ability to place our body in the right place at the right time. Power Positions exist in every range of body movements.

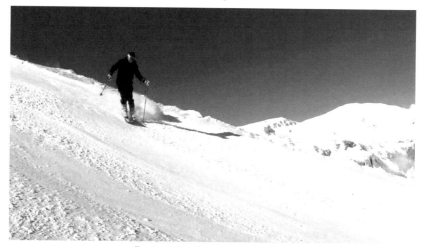

Begin skiing down a gentle slope.

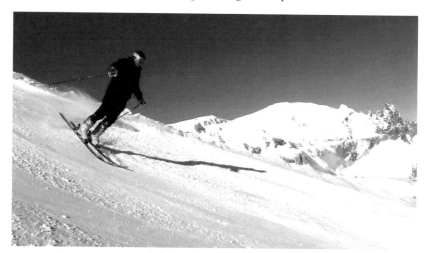

While in motion, jump up.

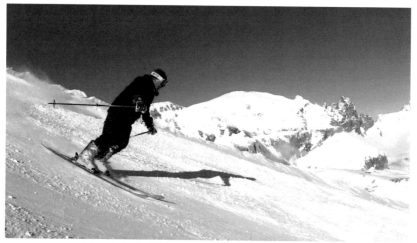

Absorb the landing and cruise into a wide radius turn.

Power

POWER POSITION TURN

●

Goal: To add downhill movement and wide turns to the Power Position for a mobile, powerful stance.

Body Position: Ski straight downhill, jump up and down three times, then make three turns.

Please refer to the ATS App for more instruction and the video demonstration of this drill.

THE POWER POSITION TURN FORCES skiers to be rhythmic, dynamic, balanced, and responsive. Even though this is a Green Circle drill, it is important to master for skiing more challenging terrain. Clients often ask how to prepare for skiing difficult terrain. I show them this drill and, if they can perform it and the three jumps between two sets of turns, I tell them they are ready to take on new challenges.

Begin skiing straight down a gentle slope. Once you're in motion, jump up—just as you did in Power Position. Recall what you learned about landing and absorbing the jump. Don't tense up and stop the compression and absorption once your skis touch the snow. Stay loose, absorb the whole landing, and spring up again.

Perform three jumps, then cruise into a wide radius turn. Perform three turns and then, if you're feeling confident, straighten out and perform three more jumps. Now make three more turns.

As you follow the jumps with turns, you'll begin to feel a new power and confidence. Your skis will feel lighter on your feet and much more responsive. This is because you are skiing in a balanced, mobile stance. Nothing can get in your way.

This drill takes confidence and commitment. Make sure you don't lose control by accelerating too quickly in the jumps. Remember to absorb the landing, using knee angulation and edge pressure in the turns to ski at a constant speed.

Mobility is the key term here. When we want to change direction or alter our skiing in some way, the most efficient method is to lift our skis. Developing a powerful stance, along with the confidence and flexibility gained from the Power Position, is an excellent way to increase your mobility. Practice this drill until you feel the power while transitioning between turning and jumping. With newfound confidence in your ability to adjust and change your rhythm, you are skiing toward the Zone of Excellence.

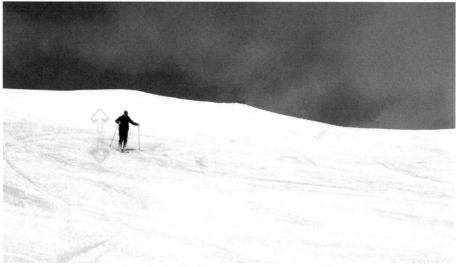

Stand tall with skis straight to pick up speed.

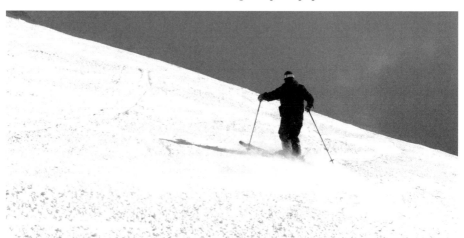

Pivot your body from the waist down and turn your skis 90 degrees to the left or right

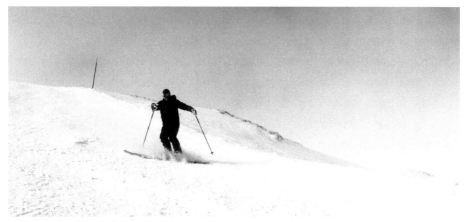

Pivot only from the waist down. Keep your body and arms facing downhill

Power

POWER SLIDE

> **Goal:** To feel a flat ski sliding in the fall line without losing control.
>
> **Body Position:** Ski straight downhill, then pivot ninety degrees and slide down the fall line.
>
> Please refer to the ATS App for more instruction and the video demonstration of this drill.

THE FIRST THIRTEEN DRILLS IN this book are designed to develop a properly balanced stance. Now, we are going to focus on developing awareness and pressuring your skis. Skis are designed for three things: sliding, edging, and carving. A sliding ski is a flat ski with no pressure or weight on the edges. An edged ski is a traversing ski; the ski isn't turning—it's transporting the skier across the hill. A carving ski is a turning ski with pressure initiated to the shovel, or front, of the ski.

The Power Slide drill focuses on a sliding ski, with no pressure on its edges. In this position, stand tall, perpendicular to the hill, while gravity pulls you.

Begin skiing down a well-groomed slope with a fair amount of pitch to it. Stand up tall and ski straight, allowing yourself to pick up some speed. Square your shoulders to the hill and focus your gaze down the fall line. Really *feel* your feet. Concentrate on your feet as the center of the ski. Once you feel as perfectly balanced and centered as possible, pivot your body from the waist down, turning your skis ninety degrees to the left or right. Be sure to pivot only from the waist down, while your upper body and arms remain facing downhill.

Check your center. Make sure your feet are equally weighted, and hold the position comfortably. If you find yourself slowing down or drifting, you're using your edges. Flatten your skis by rolling your knees and ankles away from the hill. Your path is your result. If you can slide down the fall line, you're riding a flat ski. If your edges bite into the slope, you will traverse or travel across the slope. Fine-tune your stance until you can slide down the fall line.

Once you've mastered the Power Slide, work on the Double Power Slide! In this phase, you'll learn to reverse the direction of a slide from one side to the other. Find your center and pivot from the waist down, turning your skis just as you did in Power Slide. Ski a short distance, then reverse direction and continue your Double Power Slide.

This skill is a prerequisite for entering the Zone of Excellence. Continue practicing the Power Slide and Double Power Slide until you don't have to check where your center is, and can reverse direction with ease. Remember, your path is your result. When you can Double Power Slide in the fall line, you have mastered this drill.

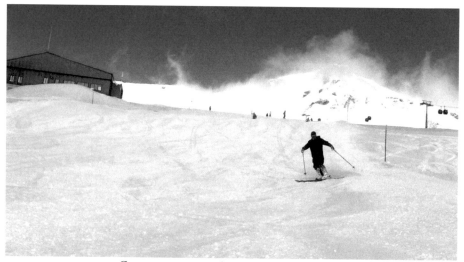

Concentrate on your feet at the center of the ski

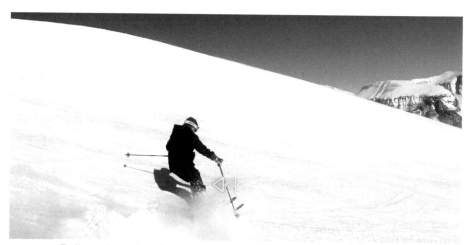

Roll your knees into the hill and turn your downhill ski edge into the snow.

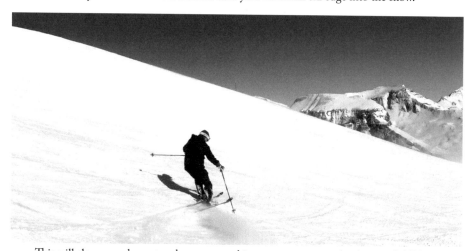

This will slow your descent and cause your skis to traverse across the slope and fall line.

Power

POWER SLIDE TO TRAVERSE

Goal: To feel the transition from a flat ski to a ski on edge.

Body Position: Three quarters of the way through a Power Slide, apply knee angulation and traverse the hill.

Please refer to the ATS App for more instruction and
the video demonstration of this drill.

MASTERY OF THE FLAT SKI is prerequisite for conquering the ski's edge. And power comes from learning a range of skills you can apply to a ski. Not only will you derive more pleasure from skiing, knowing how to ski a flat ski as well as an edged ski, but you'll gain more control and confidence. (Recall that edging is the second of the three Foundational Skills for ski control.)

Begin this drill by executing a Power Slide. As before, your upper body is relaxed, facing downhill, and your lower body is pivoted into the slide, knees and ankles adjusted to ride a flat ski. Once you're ready to traverse, apply a little knee angulation—roll your knees into the hill. As you do this, turn the downhill ski's edge into the snow, slowing your descent and causing your skis to traverse across the slope. This will bring you across the fall line.

The only difference between the Power Slide and the Power Slide to Traverse is knee angulation. Be sure you understand how this affects your centering, and how much control you can achieve just by applying pressure to your edges. On Dan's ATS II App, note the difference between the Power Slide drill and this one; you can clearly see the skier's knees rotating into the hill. Practice this drill often and work carefully with it. As you become more proficient, you'll learn the right amount of touch necessary for selective edge pressuring, which will give you the ability to apply pressure to your edges at different stages of a turn or descent. This is important in all-terrain skiing, because it gives you the flexibility to touch your edges to the snow, as well as release those edges when you want more control—a tool you'll use again and again in mountain skiing.

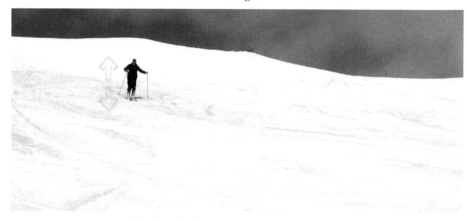

Stand tall and prepare to make a power slide.

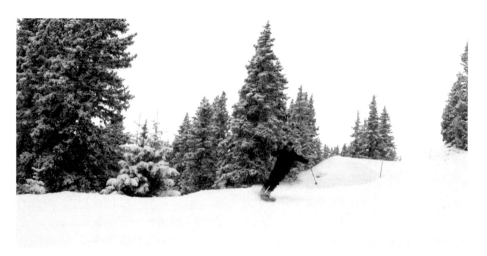

Apply knee angulation with forward pressure to your boots

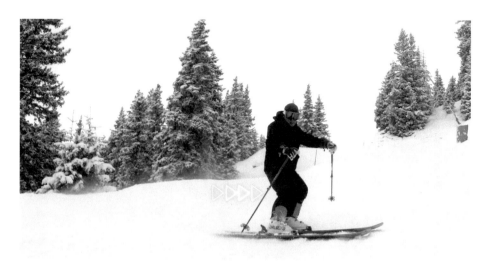

Press your shins against the tops of your boots

Power

POWER SLIDE TO CARVE

> **Goal:** To understand the transition from a flat ski to a carving ski.
> **Body Position:** Apply knee angulation and forward pressure to a Power Slide.
>
> Please refer to the ATS App for more instruction and
> the video demonstration of this drill.

THIS DRILL FOCUSES ON THE third Foundational Skill for ski control. The Power Slide to Traverse added knee angulation to the Power Slide. In order to make a turn, the Power Slide to Carve adds another subtle, yet important, movement to the Power Slide to Traverse. Begin as you have before, skiing down the slope. Keep your upper body calm, strong, and square to the slope. Be sure your arms are out in front of you and you're looking downhill.

Go into a Power Slide, then apply knee angulation with forward pressure by pressing your shins against your boots. This downward pressure will initiate carving, and your skis will turn and angle back up the slope. Knee angulation causes pressure on the ski's edge. Forward pressure on the boot puts pressure on the shovel, or tip, of the ski. This simple illustration of a carved turn demonstrates the difference between edging and carving. Do this drill in both directions. As shown in Dan's ATS II App, forward pressure and knee angulation can carve a ski with ease.

These three drills are the foundation for controlling your skis: Power Slide taught you to control a sliding ski; Power Slide to Traverse taught you to control the ski's edge; Power Slide to Carve teaches control of a carving ski, and combines the skills learned in all three.

Practice these three Foundational Skills—sliding, edging, and carving—until they are second nature. In the process, you will develop an innate sense of your center, and a calm, strong upper body. Used together, these skills and body knowledge take you into the Zone of Excellence. By mastering these skills, you become an efficient skier, receiving the maximum return for a minimal amount of energy output.

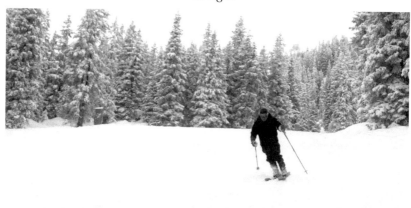

Break the run into sections

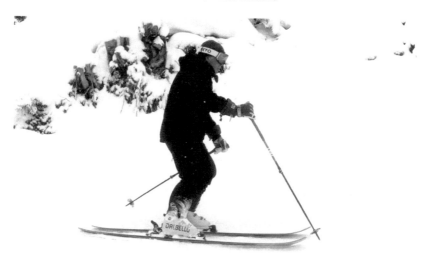

Make a series of flowing turns

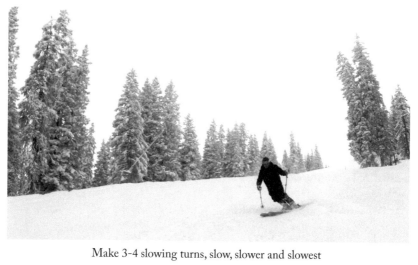

Make 3-4 slowing turns, slow, slower and slowest

Power

SLOWING AND FLOWING TURNS

■

Goal: To create the opportunity for skiers to choose when to slow down.

Body Position: Choose a run you are comfortable skiing and make a series of six to nine turns in sets of three, flowing for three turns, then slowing for three turns.

Please refer to the ATS App for more instruction and the video demonstration of this drill.

I'VE NEVER MET A SKI engineer who designed a ski to go slow—skis are designed to make a predetermined radius turn, and to accelerate. The wider skis these days are fast. Because of the increased surface area, the ski floats and glides forward, which moves the foot out in front of the hips, resulting in the skier being in the "back seat."

Attempting to slow down at the end of a turn, by pushing or bracing against the downhill ski, will stiffen the ankles, knees, and hips, causing the ski to skid and putting the skier out of balance. And if you do this with every turn, you'll never gain balance, flow, or efficiency. Turning with the purpose of slowing down will make your legs tired, and because you're skiing slowly and making short turns, you're also overturning.

Try making a series of three or four flowing turns, letting the skis flow down the fall line, then a series of slowing turns: slow, slower, then slowest. At that point, either stop, regroup, and go again, or carry on with another sequence of three to four flowing turns in the fall line, then the slowing turns again—slow, slower, and slowest—then stop.

Slowing down is an intentional strategic move while skiing. The how, where, and when of slowing down is an important decision made in advance of a run. I start each run with an intentional plan, breaking the trail down into sections. That way, I know where I'm starting, where I'm going, and where I will stop. Once I determine the sections of my route, I look for deceleration points along the way of each section. Sometimes it can be pillows of fresh snow or, in moguls, the top and downhill sides of bumps. Or I search for plateaus that will make a good target to aim for, using longer, slower arcs to check my speed.

To review: map out your run, skiing the trail in sections. Turn into the fall line making flowing turns, then as you approach your planned area to slow down, make three slowing turns—slow, slower, slowest—then exhale, smile, and repeat the flowing turns. Repeat as necessary, especially the smile.

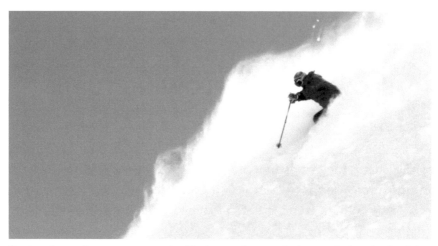

See how long of an arc you can make. The longer the turn the longer the length of stability

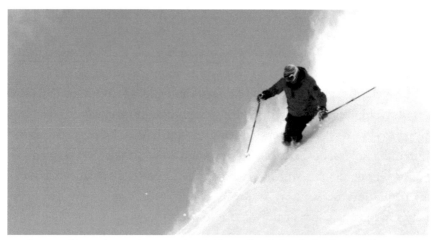

As your skis accelerate, drive your hands forward and absorb the forces of the turn.

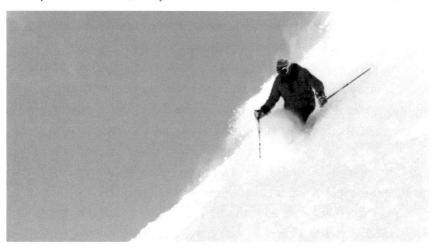

When your skis start to come across the fall line, initiate your next turn with
as short of a transition as you can

Power

LONG TURNS FOR STABILITY

> **Goal:** To experience the stability of long, arcing turns.
>
> **Body Position:** Ski an intermediate slope making long-radius turns, not allowing your skis to cross perpendicular to the fall line.
>
> Please refer to the ATS App for more instruction and the video demonstration of this drill.

NOW THAT WE UNDERSTAND HOW to slow the skis and how to let the skis flow, lets discover how to make the skis feel stable while we ride them. Ski are designed with an established turn radius, and when the ski is allowed to turn along this radius, they are stable. This is not to say they don't accelerate—but when turning down the fall line in their predetermined arc, they form a stable platform for the skier to stand on. But most skiers don't allow the skis to flow down the hill in long arcs; they tend to end the turn early, attempting to slow down and control speed.

In this drill we're going to learn to ride the ski in long, arcing turns, making short transitions between turns. What you will experience is not uncontrollable acceleration, on the contrary, you will discover a consistent speed in a stable turn, which over time will increase your confidence and efficiency while skiing.

In this drill it is important to let your skis run down the fall line, not across it. Start on a groomed intermediate slope. Point your skis down the hill, and start to turn by edging with your ankles, knees, and hips. Don't rush the turn, see how long an arc you can make. As the skis come across the fall line, initiate your next turn with as short a transition as you can, and start the new turn. Be patient, allowing the ski to find its predesigned arc. Be in your fluid athletic stance, with pressure on both skis, and allow your skis to accelerate into the fall line, driving your hands forward, sinking down to absorb the turn, then begin the new arc before the skis become perpendicular to the fall line. Make three or four turns, then stop. And repeat.

Each time you do a set of these long arcs, observe how stable the skis feel in the turn, get a sense of the speed, and begin to gain confidence that you can control both the length of the arc and the position that you stand on the ski. As you start to master this technique, you'll see how the absorption and extension of your body will dictate the length of the arc. Quick absorptions and extensions equal short turns; long, evenly paced absorptions and extensions equal long turns. When you combine this with Slowing and Flowing Turns, you are gaining mastery over your skiing and can start to explore more diverse terrain.

A REVIEW OF WHAT WE'VE LEARNED SO FAR:

BALANCE. IN THE FIRST CHAPTER, Balance, we learned about the efficient use of our body in relation to gravity. The Balance chapter also demonstrated the use of knee and hip angulation, as well as foot placement.

UPPER BODY. THE UPPER BODY chapter taught upper body positioning. The concept of isolation and separation of body parts was introduced to create a relationship between all body parts while in constant fluid motion. We learned where to focus our eyes, as well as proper hand and arm position for pole plants.

POWER. NEXT, POWER WAS INTRODUCED. We learned that a powerful stance is one that is never stagnant or rigid. Drills in this chapter illustrated how Power can be fluid and graceful, as well as explosive and dynamic. We also learned the three Foundational Skills necessary to achieve ski control: sliding, edging, and carving.

COMING UP: FLUIDITY AND AGILITY. In the next two chapters, Fluidity and Agility, the drills will take you through a range of skills, building upon the first three concepts you've learned. Pay attention to every drill, as each plays a part in working toward improving your ability for all-terrain skiing. The goal now is to add the elements of greater body awareness through isolation and separation of body parts, constant fluid motion for greater ski control, and the ability to adapt to changing terrain, conditions, speed, and situations.

As you move ahead, internalize the motions and visualize the action of the carving ski. Try to imagine what it feels like to have your body and skis working in harmony, accomplishing the goal of efficient movements to give you greater skiing control, power, fluidity, and agility. If you start to have problems with any of the drills, review previous lessons to identify your problem areas—identify the part of your body that is causing you to lose balance or control of your skis, then think about which drills you had trouble with—you will probably find a correlation between past and present problems. Repeat those drills until you have them perfected, before moving on to the next lessons. If at any point a drill stumps you, or you hit a roadblock, review the previous drills or repeat the current drill until you nail it.

ACCELERATION:
THE UNSPOKEN FEAR OF SKIERS

BEFORE WE MOVE ON, LET'S have a short conversation about acceleration, an unspoken fear among skiers. The thought sits deep in our minds: "If I go too fast, I will lose control." My goal is to change the way you view acceleration by shifting the focus from "going too fast" to staying in balance.

How many times have you looked down a slope where conditions were less than perfect, or at the entrance to a tree run that looked too narrow, and thought, "What if I end up going too fast?" This situation plays out time and time again because we fear blowing a turn or being unable to make a second turn to avoid an obstacle such as a rock, stump, or bump.

To fully grasp acceleration, we must resolve a few things. First off, skis accelerate because of a combination of engineering, technology, and materials. Secondly, when we tune our skis, waxing them and sharpening the edges, we are making the skis go faster.

Now, when you factor into the equation that most skiers fear speed, and that the skis they've purchased are designed to go fast, you have a contradiction. This fear results in physical tension, which eventually causes fatigue, errors in judgment, or an accident.

In my camps we attack this issue head-on. I tell everyone the same thing: "Skis are designed to accelerate." The purpose of turning is not to slow down, rather it's to accelerate. Turns allow us to change direction and direct the energy created by turning down the mountain in a controlled fashion.

Ultimately, skis are used as brakes. Their edges can be used as a tool to slow us down and stop. However, that is not the pure purpose of turning. The problem most skiers have is not acceleration itself, but *the lack of anticipation of acceleration*. A narrow range of balancing skills often compounds this issue. If a skier accelerates, gets going too fast, and grows fearful, they are likely to become out of balance. That might result in an unnecessarily long traverse, a need to slam on the brakes, or even a potential crash.

So, what's the trick? And how do we embrace acceleration and let go of the fear of going too fast? Anticipation of acceleration. This requires proactive body movements, which will allow the skier to stay centered and balanced over the skis as they accelerate.

Here are three examples of proactive body movements that can counter acceleration:

1) Looking ahead and down the hill. In situations where skiers are nervous, they tend to look across the hill or at the obstacle, which limits their movement into the next turn.
2) Planting the downhill pole to initiate the next turn. This will position your upper body over your skis and allow the skis to change direction while keeping your body balanced.

3) Lowering the edge angle of your skis as you enter the first turn. This will scrub unwanted speed and allow you to maneuver in tight places. It will also allow you to slide down the mountain rather than across the fall line.

If you combine all three of these tools as you enter a run, the result will be greater control, a tighter line down the mountain, and a wider range of balance. Try this for a few runs the next time you go out skiing: Ski a run you know well with the intention of only slowing down every third or fourth turn. Make two or three smooth, round turns. Allow your skis to jet out of the turn into the transition, and actively engage into the next turn, feeling the speed. Then make one turn where you hit the edges hard, skid a bit, and slow down. Repeat this series of turns. When you transform uncontrollable acceleration into the efficient use of controlled acceleration, your all-terrain skiing will take a giant leap forward.

Keep these proactive body movements in mind as we move into the Fluidity and Agility chapters of this program. These drills are sure to help you master controllable acceleration.

RHYTHM ROMANCE:
HOW TO BECOME A FLUID SKIER

FLUIDITY ADDS THE ART OF dance to the movement of skiing. Next, you'll discover how to overcome your challenges and break through to new levels of ability.

By now, you're tuned in to your body position; you have the tools, and you're learning to use them. Your free skiing is improving, and you're getting better at adapting to changes in conditions and terrain. Speed no longer scares you; rather, you're able to control it and enjoy your skiing even more. All this has been accomplished through understanding your body position and its effects on your skis.

Now it's time to add fluidity, grace, and rhythm. It's time to complement the hill with your skiing presence. In this chapter, you'll learn how to ski the mountain without letting it ski you. I define fluidity in skiing as the ability to correct body position with minor adjustments that help you stay in control. Situational skiing is the best way for skiers to discover the dance within themselves. The result will be a more elegant, fluid style of skiing.

The drills in this chapter are designed to help you accomplish a task, or body position, that enhances efficiency. The goal is to illustrate how positioning your body or skis will allow you to change direction and turn. The first drill in the Fluidity chapter, Thousand Steps, introduces the concept of selective edge pressure and how the ski can travel in an arc with constant edge pressure. The Three Edge Turns drill advances the idea that, during a turn, the ski is prepped, edged, and released while making carving turns. The Angle of Entry drill demonstrates how we position our skis down the hill to enter into a carved turn, not across the fall line. Arcing a Turn builds off the concepts introduced in the Long Turns for Stability drill from the previous chapter, and encourages body angulation and ski positioning with dynamic independent leg action. And You Go Where You Look builds upon the Look Down the Hill drill from the Upper Body chapter.

All of these drills are designed to add fluid motion to your skiing while you discover the benefits of selective edge pressure, and will help you internalize the feeling of fluidity when turning your skis and building what I call "the touch" necessary for mastering the skills in this chapter.

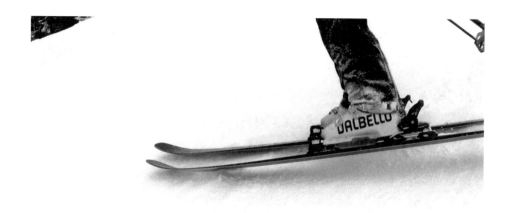

Relax, take many small light steps

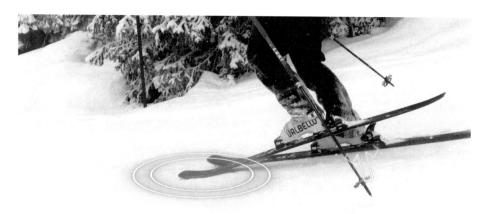

Both skis should never be on the ground at the same time

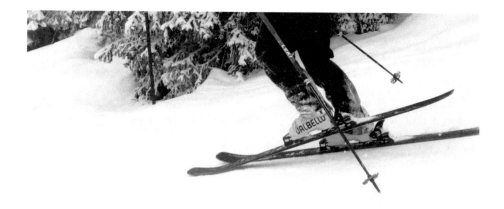

As you approach the point where you must change direction, keep making small steps

Fluidity

THOUSAND STEPS

■

> **Goal:** To establish agile, independent leg action while turning your skis.
>
> **Body Position:** Make medium to large turns on a groomed slope, making small marching steps while remaining calm and strong.
>
> Please refer to the ATS App for more instruction and
> the video demonstration of this drill.

SMALL STEPS LEAD TO BIG leaps in your skiing improvement. That's the reason for all these drills. In the Thousand Steps drill, the small steps are designed to help you identify your Frozen Zone. The Frozen Zone is the moment of realization that you've lost balance and can't move your feet. At that moment your body is out of alignment. This drill will help you identify your Frozen Zone and teach you the mobility, independent leg action, and agility necessary to overcome it.

Most skiers have problems in the belly of the turn. To correct this, we are going to make small marching steps while skiing and carving our way down the mountain. Like most drills, this exercise provides self-diagnosis and instant feedback. If at any time while making small marching steps throughout your turns, you feel stuck or unable to make steps, you are out of balance and chances are your hips are too far back behind your feet.

Choose a groomed slope you are comfortable with, beginner or intermediate. Start by gliding diagonally across the slope while making small, quick, marching steps. Focus on keeping the tips of your skis on the snow, just lifting the heels and tails of your skis. Avoid making large marching steps.

Now, start to turn while you are stepping, attempting to step through the entire arc of the turn during the transition into the new turn. Continue stepping through the entire process. Make three or four turns in this fashion. Stop, and repeat. Make any adjustments needed to be able to make steps throughout each turn. If at any time you feel unable to make the steps, adjust your body position, especially your hips, until you feel freer to move and make the steps. This exploration of correcting body position while under motion puts you inside the Breakthrough Zone, and within mastery of your skiing position. Repeat this drill until your steps are smooth and effortless. Notice how the skis travel along the radius of the turn even though they do not have constant edge pressure. This selective edge pressure, created by placing the ski on edge in a turn then lifting it as the uphill ski replaces its contact with the snow, is a powerful feeling.

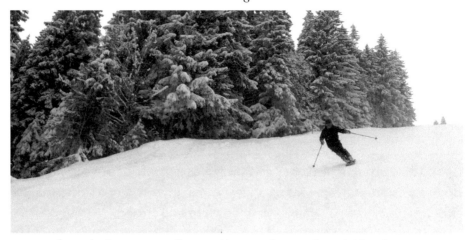

As you begin your turn, roll your ankles onto the new edge to initiate the turn

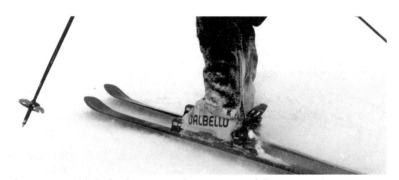

Once the turn is established, release your edge pressure and flatten your skis.

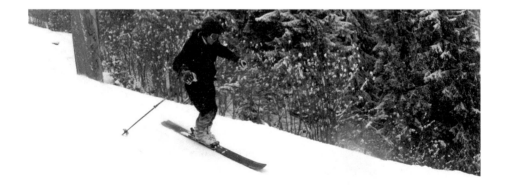

Once the skis are flat, roll them back onto their edges at the center of the turn.

Fluidity

THREE EDGE TURNS

■

> **Goal:** To build awareness of selective edge pressure and its benefits.
>
> **Body Position:** Start on a Green Circle or Blue Square groomed trail, stand tall, be calm and strong, and pressure your edges three separate times during each turn.
>
> Please refer to the ATS App for more instruction and
> the video demonstration of this drill.

NOW THAT WE'RE ON THE path to fluidity, we'll stop again to study how to expend minimal energy to achieve maximum results. Three Edge Turns is designed to further the concept of selective edge pressure. In this drill, you will focus on your ankles to create and release pressure on the skis' edges three times during one turn. Ski diagonally across the slope, rolling your ankles to initiate the turn. Once the turn is established, release the edge pressure and flatten the ski. Once the ski is flat, roll back onto the same edge in the center of the turn, then flatten the ski once again. At the tail of the turn, roll the skis back onto that edge and finish the turn. In the transition for a new turn, run a flat ski and roll the skis onto the opposite edge to initiate the new turn, flatten the skis, edge them in the center of the turn, then flatten them again, edging both skis to finish the second turn.

Once this rhythm feels natural, start to explore the length of the turns by making quick edge pressure shifts—quicker releases for short turns, longer-held edge pressure and longer flat-ski distances for longer turns. Again, this drill is illustrating that you can turn a ski without constant edge pressure, and you—the skier—can decide when and where to pressure a ski during the turn.

Three Edge Turns builds so many skills—timing of edge pressure, the slight muscle mastery of rolling your ankles, and the subtle touch of being on your edges without excessive pressure. When we talk about becoming a fluid skier, this is exactly what we're discussing—small effective moves that adjust ski performance, overall direction, and control of the skis. Your confidence for control will reach new levels because now we're not just using the word control for speed, we're using it to describe the overall descent down the mountain.

Effortless and efficient. Achieving maximum response or movement with minimal energy expenditure—that is achieving fluidity. This simple drill will take you to new heights of awareness. Your body and equipment are forming a relationship, a bond, resulting in a more fluid skiing style. This is "the touch." It feels great, doesn't it?

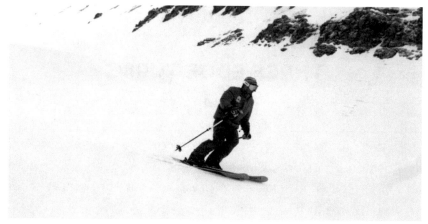

This provides momentum and gets you up to speed,
which makes it more natural to start a turn

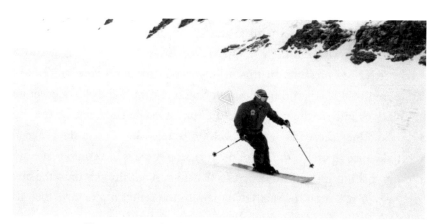

Choose your angle of entry based on the pitch of the slope

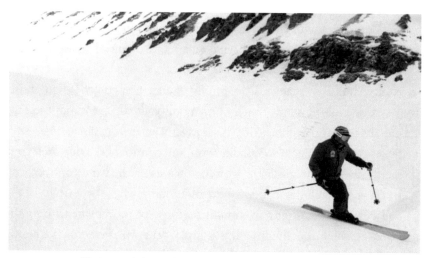

Understand the angle in which you enter into your turns

Fluidity

ANGLE OF ENTRY

∎

> **Goal:** To understand the angle in which you enter into your turns.
>
> **Body Position:** Stand tall in an athletic stance, let your skis run diagonally across the slope, choosing the beginning of your run intentionally, and begin making medium- to long-radius turns.
>
> Please refer to the ATS App for more instruction and
> the video demonstration of this drill.

THE ANGLE OF ENTRY DRILL complements several drills in previous chapters, such as Tip Hops in the Balance chapter, Downhill Hand Sweep in the Upper Body chapter, and Long Turns for Stability in the Power chapter.

We began previous drills in the Fluidity chapter by skiing diagonally across the hill. There are many advantages to starting your run in this fashion. First of all, beginning a run diagonally provides momentum and gets you up to skiing speed, so it's more natural to initiate a turn. Second, by starting in a diagonal direction, your skis will have an easier time entering the fall line. As in Long Turns for Stability, where we allowed the skis to find their predetermined radius, this drill emphasizes the point of entry into a turn that is most efficient.

By making an intentional decision to choose your angle of entry into a turn, you are mentally starting to understand the many aspects of turning. Physically, you are purposely aiming your skis to a certain part of the slope. Emotionally, you are choosing the moment and situation in which you find yourself. Skiing is not one-size-turn-fits-all; you need to set an intention, purpose, and emotional commitment to the choices you are making while skiing.

I choose my angle of entry based on the pitch of the slope. On Green Circle slopes, my skis ride more directly down the fall line; on Blue Square trails, I aim slightly off the fall line; on Black Diamonds, I ski halfway between perpendicular and straight down. Up on the big steep faces, depending on the width of the slope, I drop the tips of my skis just from perpendicular to the slope, and begin to move into the turn. Mastering Angle of Entry is another milestone on the trail to the Zone of Excellence.

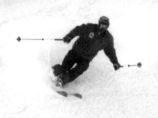

Visualize yourself arcing turns in a smooth fluid fashion down the slope

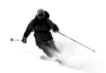

Visualize yourself arcing turns in a smooth fluid fashion down the slope

The length of the arcs of the turns you want to make in different section

Fluidity

ARCING A TURN

■

The Goal: To start seeing terrain from the perspective of applying the skills you're learning to varying conditions.
Body Position: Look down the slope, visualizing yourself skiing it. Identify the different sections of the trail, and the radius of the turns that work best for each section, then push off and implement your plan.
Please refer to the ATS App for more instruction and the video demonstration of this drill.

NOW WE'RE MOVING INTO THE part of *All-Terrain Skiing* that I refer to as Applied Technique. As your skills build, you can start to apply them to every run with intention and purpose. Fluidity isn't just smooth skiing—it's being able to react quickly, and with confidence. That's where Arcing a Turn comes in. This drill tests your reactions and balance, teaching you to achieve fluid motion through the isolation and separation of body parts. It's also a great energy drill! Its purpose is to orchestrate the entire gamut of body dynamics—working with poles, shoulders, arms, hands, hips, legs, knees, edges, boots, and feet.

Now that you understand selective edge pressure, as well as how the arc of the turn creates a stable platform, start mixing up the flow of your turns, from short radius to long radius. This will add control to your skiing and broaden your decision making as far as where you go and why. Often, the slope that starts off perfect for medium radius turns narrows in the midsection, requiring shorter turns, and opens up at the bottom, ideal for wide-open, arcing turns.

Now that you're in the Breakthrough Zone, discovering the fluidity of skiing, stand on top of your favorite challenging ski run. Look down the fall line and see yourself arcing turns in a smooth, fluid fashion down the slope. Identify the different sections of the trail that call for flowing and slowing. Visualize the length the arc for ideal turns in that section. Now push off and ski your predetermined plan, mixing up the lengths of your arcs and the pace of your turns. This drill creates space for you to ski in your own style down slope, with anticipation of reading the terrain and adapting what you've learned so far in this book. The beauty is, you can do this drill countless times during your ski day, on any run you choose.

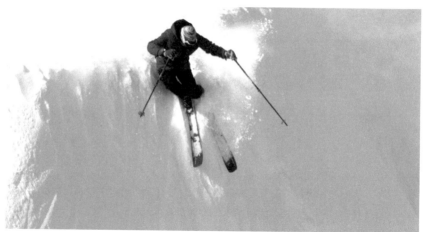

Break the slope into sections

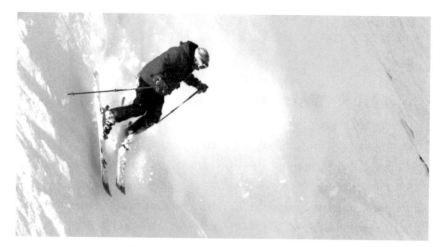

Note the best route around the obstacles

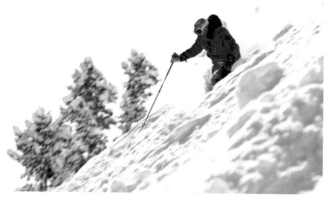

Keep your eyes looking down the fall line adjusting the arc of your turns as needed and keeping your eyes focused on the route you determined

70

Fluidity

YOU GO WHERE YOU LOOK

Goal: To make visual assessment an active part of skiing.

Body Position: Study the run, visualize your path, identify obstacles, and look away from them to the path that provides the most fluid descent.

Please refer to the ATS App for more instruction and
the video demonstration of this drill.

SKIING IS A TOTAL-BODY EXPERIENCE, which is why in this program we deal with every aspect of how athletes perform, including the often-overlooked aspect of the eyes. The first drill in the Upper Body chapter, Look Down the Hill, highlights the importance our head and eyes play in our athletic activities, and how to get the eyes to focus on looking down, rather than across the hill. Now we are going to elevate that concept to the next level in order to increase our fluid motion. Our eyes play a critical part in how we interpret the terrain we are skiing. How we see it will determine how we ski it. This is important—what we see, how we see it, and how we react to it all matter while skiing. Some skiers balk at obstacles without realizing how that reaction affects their performance.

You go where you look, so look where you want to go. Look away from obstacles, so you don't go straight for them. Throughout this book, I've been discussing the importance of the fall line, as that is where gravity pulls us. Therefore, it makes sense that we want to look down the fall line, as that is our primary focus. Obstacles not in the fall line are not our concern. So, if there is a rock wall on the right or a big tree on the left, look between them. But what if there is an obstacle in the fall line? A rock, bump, or stump—how do we ski safely around it?

In the Arcing a Turn drill we discussed visualizing your run, breaking the trail down into sections, and designing the radius of your turns per the different sections of the slope. This drill is a complement to that one because, understanding that "we go where we look, so look where you want to go," we can look down the fall line, see the obstacle, and look away from it to the open space beside it, and flow into that, around the obstruction, without stopping or getting stuck.

To begin, while standing on top of a run, look down the fall line and mentally break the slope up into sections, noting obstacles and the best route around them. Then look for visual landmarks that will let you know when you're approaching the obstacle. Tell yourself where you're going to look when you get to that section of the run. During the run, gaze down the fall line, adjusting the arc of your turns as needed. When you get to the landmark, focus your eyes on the way around the obstacle, and adjust your route as needed.

This will take practice. Often, the first time down a run, I'll put in a check turn or a power slide well above an obstacle, just to ensure all is well. But over time, as I come back to that run, I am determined to take it in stride and ski around it while maintaining my fluid ski run.

A natural place to practice this technique is on an intermediate mogul run or glades. Analyze the fall line, identify the obstacles, visualize a plan, and go. Ski the same line again and again until it becomes second nature. Then move on to another trail, and repeat until you master that one as well.

THE BREAKTHROUGH ZONE

CONGRATULATIONS ON MAKING IT THIS far in the program. If you are mastering the drills and skills, no matter how silly or strange they may seem, I'm confident you are changing your paradigm not only for *how* you ski but *where* you ski. Welcome to the Breakthrough Zone. Every year people come to my camps and clinics with the same goal: they want to break through to the next level in their skiing. Following the concepts of this program, they start to become all-terrain skiers. Over the years I have discovered that the best way to inject skiing with new energy and skill is to take a step back from your current skiing comfort zone and enter the Breakthrough Zone. The key to that is different for everyone, and may include moguls, trees, control, speed, or hard-packed snow.

The Breakthrough Zone (BZ) is the equivalent of reprogramming your computer's hard drive. In the BZ, we update and reboot our physical and mental approach to skiing. Many of the ruts we fall into have to do with who, where, and when we ski, so the BZ starts with how and when you arrive at the mountain, with whom you ski, and much more. Remember, BZ skiing is all about busting wide open into new realms of experience.

Matching motivations. It's important to find ski friends who match your motivation for improving. You don't have to ski all day with these people, but plan on at least two hours of your ski day. This is very helpful for making progress.

Skills and drills time. You must always remain motivated enough to practice. If you want to be better at steeps, you need to focus on the basics—upper body, pole planting, and quick edge-to-edge transitions. Or maybe bumps are your thing. If so, you must be willing to start on medium-grade bumps and build up to the steep, rad lines. This is going to require practice, time, and patience, once again for two or more hours a day.

Turn "Oh No" into "Oh Yeah." We're all driven by some form of inner voice. It's best to flip the switch of this conversation into positive, reinforcing language, such as: "I can. I will. I am progressing. It's going to happen. There is progress happening here!"

Visualization. Skiing is a visual sport as much as it is physical. Find images and videos of other skiers who model your goals. Watch them, embed the images in your memory, and visualize them as you ski. The *All-Terrain Skiing II* Dan's ATS II App is another effective tool to help you visualize.

Burn to learn. Remember, we all fall. Falling is not a negative experience, but a learning experience if you think about it correctly. If you are going to push past your limits, you're likely going to have a few yard sales along the way. That's fine! Just part of the process. Never stop learning! Explore the possibilities of all-terrain skiing and expanding your horizons. As your confidence grows, so will your adventures. Be safe. Be smart. Be bold in your exploration of the Breakthrough Zone, and go for it!

Agility is the result of honing a sharp sense of movement. An agile skier can go wherever they please, most often with grace. An agile skier flows so beautifully, they appear to float above the snow, always seeking the path of least resistance. Since fluidity adds the art of dance to skiing, agility allows skiers to dance on any part of the mountain they desire, in just about any conditions. The goal is to operate in the Zone of Excellence.

Joseph Campbell, the author of several books on hero stories, wrote, "The best things cannot be told, because they transcend thought. The second best are misunderstood because they are the thoughts that are supposed to refer to that which cannot be thought about. The third best are what we talk about." In other words, the ultimate ski run has no translation from experience to explanation. My friend Peter Gardiner once described my smile in a skiing photograph as "sublime." Case in point.

In 1991, I took a ski trip to Slovenia (then called Yugoslavia). Our journey began in Kanine, a beautiful, small ski area on the Italian border. The summit station was surrounded by mountain peaks that hovered 1,500 to 2,000 feet above us. The slopes were steep and covered with a combination of cliffs, narrow shoots, and wide-open spaces—a perfect place to ski.

The problem was, the descent was much different from the climb. We were sure of the snow conditions, but unsure of our way through the rocks below. Our cameraman, Tom Day, set up across the valley and yelled, "Camera rolling!" via radio. In the excitement and anticipation of my first turn, I dropped one of my ski poles, and it tumbled down the steep face and out of sight.

Without hesitation, I jumped in and started skiing the 50 degree face with only one pole. After that, my memory is vague. I remember moving snow following my every turn; I remember entering the cliff band with a constant speed and unwavering confidence in my ability. Then, I remember seeing a way through the rocks and off a cliff. The landing and the turns to the bottom were nothing but a sense of freedom, power, and my "sublime" internal smile.

Months later, watching the film, I had an out-of-body experience. I remembered being there and knew I had skied it, but noticed so many details I'd forgotten. That's when I realized—when operating in the Zone of Excellence, the mind and body act as one, allowing you to perform extraordinary feats.

The discussion, drills, and skills in this final chapter of the book center around developing an instinctive reaction within yourself. The Shorten Your Transitions drill will increase your stability; Uphill Ski Pressure will develop more control on the steeps and powder. Dropping In and Settling In will set the standard for calming your nerves by providing strategy and tactics for skiing challenging terrain. Mind Over Mogul and Nonstop Skiing will help you find the path of least resistance. The Joy of Skiing ties the whole package together and gives you the time and freedom to experience the Zone of Excellence.

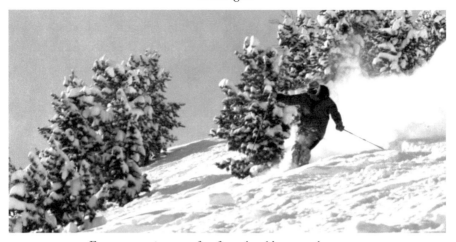

Focus on moving your feet from the old turn to the new as
quickly and efficiently as you can.

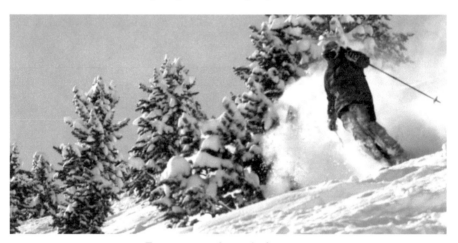

Experiment with your body position:

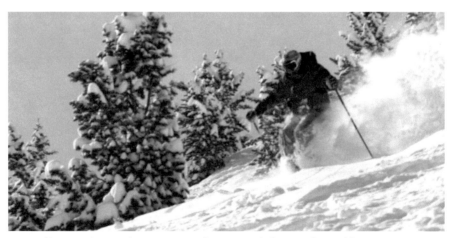

Pay attention to what movements keep you in balance and in stable position.
Incorporate those into your daily skiing.

Agility

SHORTEN YOUR TRANSITIONS

■

> **Goal:** To ski your favorite run, making six to eight turns with a focus on shortening your transitions.
>
> **Body Position:** Experiment with different body movements during your transition in order to discover the most balanced and efficient ways to enter into the next turn.
>
> Please refer to the ATS App for more instruction and
> the video demonstration of this drill.

BY NOW YOU'VE BECOME MORE aware of how to use pressure with your skis and boots. You know many types of turns and how to use your skis to control movement and direction. In skiing, we spend so much time talking about turning and all the dynamics that go along with it, but very little time talking about what to do between turns—the transitions.

I like to describe transitions as the time and space between notes of music. For me, the transitions between turns represent freedom in a time and space where my whole world slows down. I like to think about how the purpose of turning is to enter the transition.

If the turn is stable, a transition may be unstable for a few reasons: Since skis are designed to turn, a flat, unedged ski is not a stable platform. The wider the ski, the more potential the ski has to wobble or float during the transition. And because of the wide waist of modern skis, the ski can accelerate due to the amount of surface area exposed to the snow, moving the foot in front of the hip during the transition and causing the skier to be out of balance as they enter the new turn.

The key to avoiding all this is to shorten the transitions between turns, getting back to a stable stance as quickly as possible upon exiting the turn. Hesitation is acceleration, so move into the new turn quickly and deliberately. Therefore, it is very important not to attempt to slow down in the lower third of the turn; rather, you want to release the pressure on the ski in the last phase of turn. You can release the pressure of the ski by moving your hips forward, releasing pressure on your legs, feet, and ultimately the edges of your skis, entering the transition with the intention of getting to the new edge of the new turn as fast as possible. The transition allows the skier just enough time to realign their body over their feet and skis, and from this power position enter the new turn calm and strong, fluid and loose.

So, in this simple drill, ski with a focus of making quick transitions between turns.

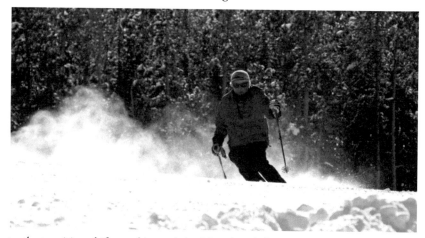

As you enter the transition, shift your hips and shoulders downhill as you extend your hand for the next pole plant

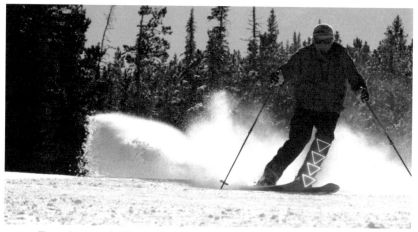

Extend your uphill leg and stand on the uphill ski to release the pressure from your downhill ski.

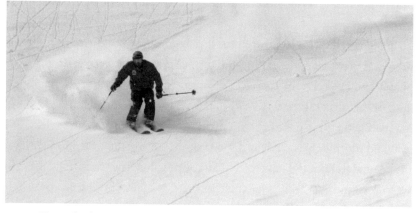

Enter the Angle of Entry and roll onto the new edges in the next turn

Agility

UPHILL SKI PRESSURE

> **Goal:** To master a deceleration technique for the steep and deep.
>
> **Body Position:** In the lower third of the turn, pressure the uphill ski prior to the transition into the next turn.
>
> Please refer to the ATS App for more instruction and the video demonstration of this drill.

AGILE SKIERS CAN CHANGE RHYTHM and direction while skiing at a constant speed. The most challenging aspect of skiing is to maintain composure while focusing on the task. Uphill Ski Pressure allows the skier to decelerate at the end of a turn in deep powder or on steeps, and provides a stable platform for moving through the transition in challenging terrain while entering a new turn. This drill requires you to handle acceleration, dynamic motion, isolation and separation of body parts, and knee angulation for edge pressure.

Start by choosing the length of your turns on a wide-open slope. Now, as you exit the belly of the turn and enter the lower third phase of the turn, pressure your uphill ski by standing up on it to release pressure on your downhill ski.

In the majority of our turns, we put 60 to 70 percent of our weight on the downhill ski. We have been taught that more pressure on the downhill ski equals more control. Therefore, many skiers over pressure the downhill ski in the lower third of the turn, in search of control. If the conditions are firm or icy, there is belief that more edge pressure will control speed. However, over pressuring the downhill ski causes the lower leg to stiffen, which pushes away from the hill. Thus, the ski can accelerate.

So, what is the fix? Pressure the uphill ski. This accomplishes the following: it moves the uphill leg into position under your hips; it releases the pressure on the downhill ski, which will eliminate unwanted acceleration; and it narrows your stance, which provides a wider platform and more stability because the skis are closer together with the total width of both skis acting as one, rather than two separate platforms. The good news—this is not difficult to accomplish. Choose the length of your arc and begin down the fall line. As you exit the belly of a turn, stand up on your uphill leg. This will lengthen your uphill leg and release pressure on the downhill ski, at the same time aligning your hips over your feet.

This is the foundation for Big Mountain Skiing, so spend some time mastering this drill.

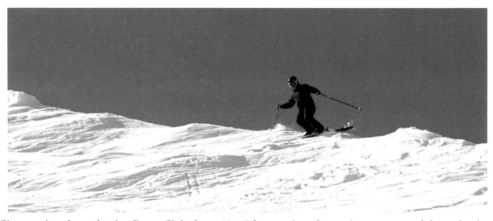

Ski over the edge and either Power Slide down 10-15 feet or take a diagonal traverse in and down the slope.

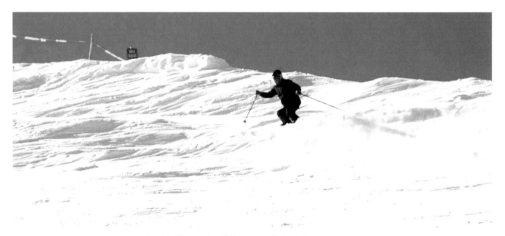

Look down the fall line and visualize your run

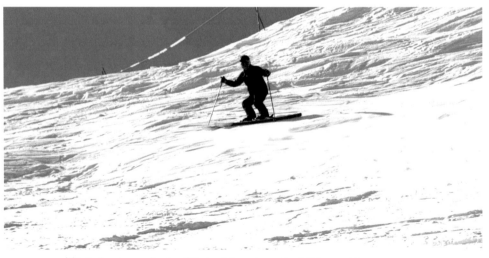

Think about your Angle of Entry. Move down the fall line and into your turn.

Agility

DROPPING IN AND SETTLING IN

> **Goal:** To form the habit of dropping directly into the run, then stopping and taking the time to prepare for success.
> **Body Position:** Be the first one off the drop, in order to settle in, choose your line, visualize that line, and then go for it.
> Please refer to the ATS App for more instruction and the video demonstration of this drill.

IT IS NORMAL TO BE nervous or unsure when skiing. Conditions, situations, and slope pitch all come into play, not to mention the sometimes not-so-helpful chatter of fellow skiers at the top of a run, commenting on what they would or wouldn't do. Know that you are not alone in the constant battle of nerves on the mountain.

At this point in the All-Terrain Skiing program, your skills are increasing. Your technique and understanding of body movements, as well as visualization and application of these skills, are all making you a better skier. Now is the time to really take control of this process to set yourself up for success on more difficult runs. To accomplish this, start to separate yourself from the crowd by dropping into mogul runs, glades, and steep pitches first. Notice I said drop in, not ski the entire run.

Here is my approach—ski over the edge or enter the slope in the following manner: either power slide down ten to fifteen feet, or take a diagonal traverse in and down the slope, then stop. Take a deep breath, shaking out any tension. Look down the fall line and visualize your run. Identify sections of the run, looking for obstacles and thinking about your arcing turns. When you're ready, push off and nail it.

The concept behind Dropping In and Settling In builds confidence. Everything will look different once you are off the cornice or over the edge of the ridge. It won't look as steep, and you can use the skills you learned earlier to power slide down into a traverse or look away from an obstruction. By dropping in and settling in, you are taking the safe route—this will start to calm your nerves, which will enhance your performance.

This is an important habit. It reinforces so much of what is in this program. Drop into it—look down the hill, not across it. Think about your angle of entry, move down the fall line and into your turn, reaching with your pole plants and enjoying the ride!

81

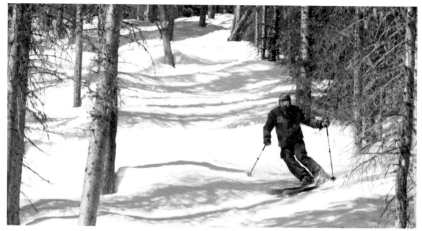

Pressure your uphill ski at the end of the turn

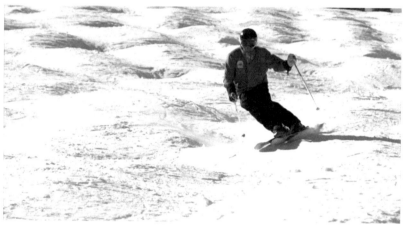

Use your pole point for your pole plant while keeping your eyes downhill. You go where you look, so look where you want to go.

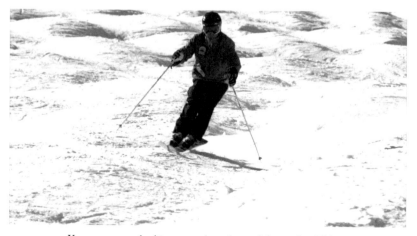

Keep your eyes looking past obstacles and down the fall line

MIND OVER MOGUL

> **Goal:** To find your own path through the moguls.
> **Body Position:** Ski in a corridor throughout a mogul run.
> Please refer to the ATS App for more instruction and
> the video demonstration of this drill.

WHEN I WAS A KID, my older brother told me, "Ski the bumps as fast as you can until you fall, then pick yourself up and do it again. Pretty soon, you'll be skiing top to bottom. Fast will seem normal, and recoveries will be no big deal." I took his advice, and it worked! But I was a kid, able to bounce and bend in a lot of directions that would be impossible for me today.

Mind Over Mogul is rooted in this philosophy, but tamer. The goal of this drill is to *ski within a confined space*. This will force you to deal with every obstacle in your path.

I like to ski in corridors where I am forced to make turns. Having boundaries provides me with the focus of where to look and when to turn, and forces me to find a constant speed. When you add moguls, the game really gets interesting. Begin skiing down a mogul field. Find your Angle of Entry, use Uphill Ski Pressure at the end of the turn, recall your Pole Point, Look Down the Hill while remembering that You Go Where You Look, so look where you want to go. This drill is called Mind Over Mogul because, when you apply the skills outlined in this program, the moguls won't matter!

Make six to eight turns; stop, regroup, and go again. Ski as wide as you like until you have no problem choosing where to turn. As you gain confidence, shorten your traverse but commit to a certain space and defined width. As you progress, bring your commitment level higher by shortening the traverse until you are skiing the fall line. This drill will build agility and identify the path of least resistance. You will notice that the moguls are less intimidating because you're learning where to turn.

On Dan's ATS II App, you can see the path of least resistance. Remember to keep looking down the fall line, past any intimidating obstacles. Mind Over Mogul is great practice for all-terrain skiing.

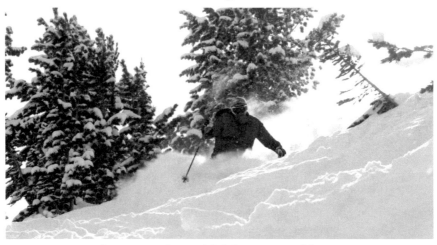

Let your mind go, and feel the sensation of skiing

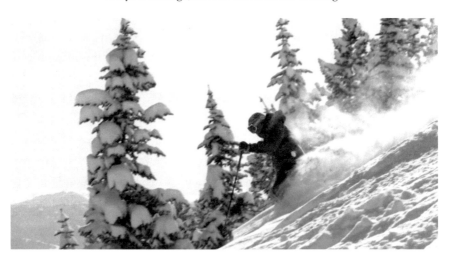

Be a passenger along for the ride

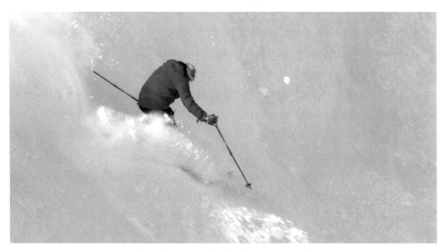

Breathe in speed and relax your mind

NONSTOP SKIING

> **Goal:** To experience changing terrain, conditions, and speed with confidence in your skillset.
>
> **Body Position:** Ski nonstop from the lift for three or more runs in a row.
>
> Please refer to the ATS App for more instruction and
> the video demonstration of this drill.

MY GRANDFATHER USED TO TELL me this story over and over when I was a child: "There was a man walking down Beacon Street in Boston, carrying a trumpet case"—he would begin, pause, and look at me like granddads do, then continue—"when a boy came up to him and asked, 'Excuse me, mister. Do you know how to get to Symphony Hall?' The man replied, *'Practice*, son, *practice!'*"

That story says it all. Skiers of all ages have asked me, "How did you get so good?" or "When did it all come together?" The truth is, it's all about mileage, laps, and vertical feet—be the first one on the lift, last one off, as often as you can. Nonstop Skiing is about getting your ski boots to feel as comfortable and natural as your favorite sneakers.

Ski top to bottom for two or three runs, nonstop. Let your mind go, and feel the sensation of skiing. Be a passenger along for the ride. Marvel at the performance of your skis and body working as one. Breathe in the speed, and relax your mind. Nonstop Skiing is the best way to build confidence and measure your ability to ski within the Zone of Excellence. You must experience your body's instinctive reactions—and learn to trust those reactions. Skiing will then become muscle memory. This drill is the combination of the whole package. The way to form muscle memory is by repeating every motion, skill, and drill in this book. As your muscle memory develops, so will your ability. Ski within your Zone of Excellence. It's only as large as you make it, so practice, practice, practice! Your Zone will grow larger as you become a better skier.

Skiing is about freedom, the force of a turn, the power of the ski edging, the dynamic motion of your body responding to the slope, and your mind awakening to speed. Skiing will not only make you a better skier, but a more fulfilled human being too. The mountains are your playground. Express yourself. Bring your style, and enjoy Nonstop Skiing. To paraphrase Campbell, the ultimate ski run has no translation from experience to words. So live it, love it, and ski it!

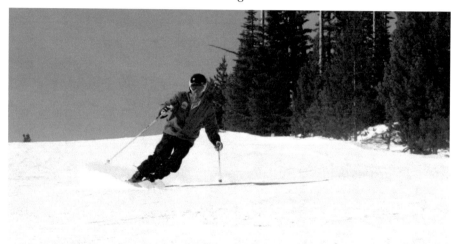

Clear your mind of any preconceptions about how to ski

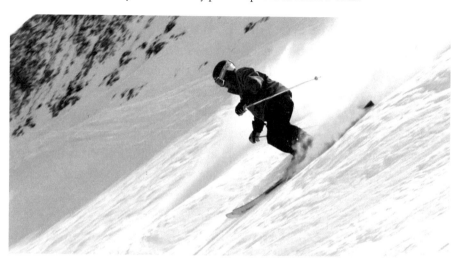

Do not focus on performance

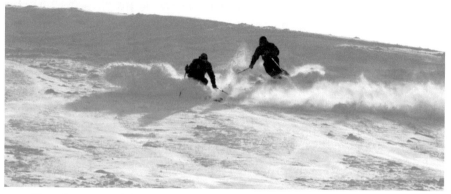

Try to have so much fun other people notice. You will help spread the joy of skiing

THE JOY OF SKIING

> **Goal:** To lose the need to improve; relax, smile, and find joy in your skiing.
>
> **Body Position:** Ski your favorite runs, creating fun, flowing turns while focusing on the here and now.
>
> Please refer to the ATS App for more instruction and the video demonstration of this drill.

YOU HAVE REACHED THE MAIN objective of this book—to inject joy into your skiing. I like to remind my clients at camps and clinics that focusing on performance can ruin a good day of skiing, and I encourage skiers not to let this happen. As our ski level increases, so should our joy. Skiing is such as great sport because we can do it long into old age. Skiing is about position, not strength. So when we obtain the proper stance and efficiency of motion, mixed with breathing and knowing where to look, paradise can be found on every run.

The goal of this drill is not to focus on performance, but to connect with the feelings skiing stirs within you. So, go and ski your favorite runs, multiple times in a row. Look around at the views, enjoy the people you are with, and take time to appreciate the Joy of Skiing. Search for the forces you feel while making a turn, the emotions you experience in the transition of the turn, the thrill of gliding on, over, and through snow, and smile. See your improvements, let go of the stumbles and bumbles, and move with freedom down the mountainside. Create a rhythm; make your skiing look like a dance full of grace and energy.

Try to have so much fun that other people take notice. You will be spreading gospels about the root reasons of why we ski—to find joy on a winter day in the mountains.

ARTICLES

I wrote these articles for the Montana newspaper, *Explore Big Sky*. I hope they will entertain and inspire you in your quest for excellence in all-terrain skiing.

Start Your Day with the Morning Glide

THE MORNING GLIDE IS HOW I refer to the first run of the day. It's simply a run to welcome the day, feel the chill in the air, and gain a sense of the snow conditions under my skis. It's a chance to say "Hello" to the day and to my body as I glide down the mountainside. I'm not trying to over-glorify the scene, just set the stage for the day.

On the first run of the morning, I do the following to set up for a day of great skiing:

Never overthink the first run. It's a judgment-free run and it's not about performance. Regardless of the conditions—firm, soft, powder, groomed—the goal is to just glide. While gliding, make big, long, sweeping turns and resist the urge to carve and accelerate. Just feel the day, find a rhythm, and breathe in the morning air.

When it comes to your ski boots, leave them a bit loose to start with. Let your foot work its way into the liner. Keeping the boots slightly loose will also enhance the blood flow to your feet, which will keep them warmer and allow them to be more reactive as the day progresses. The best practice for boots is to buckle them tighter throughout the day, but don't over-tighten them and cut off circulation. Many people crank their boots up tight and unbuckle them between runs. This is counterproductive. If you're having trouble getting a comfortable fit, see a boot fitter right away.

The main goal on the morning glide is to wake up your senses. Wave your arms, twist your torso, flex your knees deeply in the turns, and extend way up in the transitions. This is your morning stretch, a meditative flowing yoga as you glide down the slope. Often, if I feel stiff or sore in my lower back, or maybe my hamstrings are tight, I'll stop and stretch on the side of the hill, concentrating on the specific areas of my body that are asking for attention. I tend to stop a few more times than normal on the opening run of the day, just to remind myself not to rush, and to ensure this is a good, solid warm-up run. There's a lot of pressure, especially on the good snow days, to hurry and grab as much of the fresh snow as possible. I fully understand that. It's the case on any given day when fresh tracks are a premium. I select slopes that have the good snow but are wide open, so my turns can flow and I have space to focus on my breathing and movement. It's on these days when you might be skiing longer distances than normal, trying to keep up with the pack. When this happens, focus even more on breathing and lengthening your turn, as this conserves energy and allows you to lose the vertical, so you can keep up.

The morning glide for me is my time, my pace, and it creates the dynamic that sets up the entire day. It's as important to\me as the first cup of coffee. Often it feels so good I'll head right back to the top to do it all over again. And as each run gains momentum throughout the day, I start to rev up performance, increase speed, tighten up the turns, set the edges, and enjoy a full day on the hill.

Rhythm Romance: How to Become a Fluid Skier

WATCHING A GREAT SKIER IS like watching a live dance or theatrical performance. There is a lightness and a touch to their movements, each of which is accented by the constant fluid motion of energy.

In skiing, fluidity is the point where dynamic tension no longer limits motion. Rather, the skier's motion is innate and instinctive, happening in anticipation of the terrain, not in reaction. Fluidity adds the art of dance to the movement of skiing.

How do you become a fluid skier? Situational skiing is the best way to find the dance within yourself. This means constantly readjusting your body position to stay in control.

It doesn't mean tackling the most challenging terrain you're able to get down, which is how many skiers judge themselves. They wear the runs they've skied like badges of honor, defining their day by what and where they skied. This is all fine; however, if your chosen terrain causes you to ski with dynamic tension, you won't ski fluidly.

If someday you want to dance down a steep or bumpy run, you need to step back and relax on terrain you can move confidently through, rather than just survive. The result will be a more fluid style.

As I often tell students in my clinics, the best way to break through on skis is to pick a run you can master and ski it again and again—maybe five or six times in a row—taking roughly the same line each time. This will help you build confidence and discover how to anticipate the terrain rather than react to it. It's why racers train on the same course throughout a day. The repetition allows you to relax and let your body take over. You'll release the dynamic tension you've been holding and move with more dynamic motion.

Being relaxed like this also helps you tune into your body position. You will start instinctively understanding how your skis feel and react in certain situations, and how to use them. You'll also start naturally anticipating changes in conditions and terrain. Speed will no longer scare you; rather, you'll be able to control and enjoy it.

As you begin mastering terrain, you'll end up trying out different body positions. Through this experimentation, you'll develop new ways to change direction and turn your skis in a wider range of motion. Just watching someone who moves like this is a delight—experiencing it for yourself is transformative. In time you'll begin skiing the mountain instead of letting it ski you.

Deceleration Lives in the Future

MASTERING THE DRILLS AND SKILLS in this program will help you transition from the fear of acceleration into the realm of controllable acceleration. And now, to finish that concept, try to think about acceleration as something that lives out in front of you down the slope. Here is what I mean.

Many skiers try to slow down each turn they make because they are living under the delusion that the purpose of turning is deceleration. Skis are not intended to slow you down. I've never met a ski engineer who has designed a ski to go slow. Skis are designed to make a predetermined radius of a turn, and to accelerate. Each company has its theory of what materials make up the best-flexing ski, both tips to tail and torsional. Some are softer to absorb the energy created—they flex and dampen, which allows them to slow down easier. Others, like race skis, are stiff for pure acceleration. The wider skis these days are fast because of the increased surface area—the ski floats and glides forward, free of the friction of being dragged down in the snow.

If you turn with the purpose of slowing down every turn, my guess is your legs feel tired by midmorning or midday, and because you are skiing slow and making short turns, you are overturning during your descent. This is not only inefficient, but exhausting.

Deceleration lives in the future. It is too late to slow down in the turn you are making, and here's why: when a skier attempts to slow down at the end of their turn by pushing or bracing against the downhill ski, this action stiffens the ankle, knee, and hip, causing the ski to skid and putting the skier out of balance. If you do this every turn, you'll never gain balance, flow, or efficiency.

So how do we slow down the technology we have invested in? I spend a lot of time in my camps and clinics convincing skiers that, with a slight increase in speed and a mapped-out route, you can ski efficiently, save energy, and have more control. The result will be a longer, more enjoyable ski day, and eventually you will expand your mastery of the mountain.

Slowing down is an intentional strategic move while skiing, and the how, where, and when is an important decision made in advance of a run. I start each run with an intentional plan, and break the trail down into sections. That way I know where I am starting, where I am going, and where I will stop. Once I determine the different sections of the route, I look for deceleration points along the way of each section. Sometimes it can be pillows of fresh snow or, in moguls, the top and downhill sides of bumps, or I search for plateaus that make a good target to aim at, and make longer, slower arcs.

The key is to not slow down every turn; rather, ski three or four turns, letting the skis flow down the fall line, and then slow down over a series of turns. I call these my "slowing turns." In other words, I'll ski three or four turns, then make three slowing turns that are slow, slower, and slowest. At that point I'll either stop, regroup, and go again, or I'll carry on with another sequence of three to four turns in the fall line, and then make my slowing turns—slow, slower, slowest, and stop.

This is what I mean when I say deceleration lives in the future. If you want to slow down, turn. When you release the energy of a turning ski and enter a new turn, you can gain control and slow down while remaining in balance.

You can experiment with this on different slope angles. Start on your favorite Blue Square groomer run and, once you feel comfortable, venture out onto a steep pitch, or off into the trees and powder.

It is important to remember, when I make my series of slowing turns, I compress and extend more—I'm not static. The more I move up and down, the more I can control the pacing of my skis and speed.

The slowing turns commit skiers to slowing down in the future because they release the turn they are in and enter the new turn with more motion, which absorbs energy. As control is gained, speed is dissipated over a series of turns.

So as a review, map out your run and ski it in sections. Remind yourself that decelerations live in the future, and it is too late to slow down in the turn you are making. Then head down the slope and turn in the fall line. As you enter one of your planned areas to slow down, make your three slowing turns—slow, slower, slowest. Stop, smile, and continue.

Strategy and Tactics Trump Technique

MANY SKIERS ARE FOCUSED ON their technique; they want to improve and firmly believe that if the technique is mastered, they can then tackle more difficult terrain. But these skiers are missing two key elements of the sport: strategy and tactics.

What do I mean by strategy and tactics? Well, to simplify the statement, what is your plan? When looking down a mogul field, glades, powder slope, or chute I would argue an intermediate skier can enjoy these types of runs with strong strategy and focused tactics on where to go and why to go there. In other words, having a purpose and moving in the direction of that purpose is more powerful than technique.

At my camps and clinics, I've been able to take skiers of all abilities into incredible terrain, incredible powder runs, through breath-taking scenery, and often their technique is far from perfect. This is always accomplished through planning, having a strategy for where and how to enter a slope, and having the tactics of building confidence in the simple skills of traversing, stopping, and safely changing direction.

Let's start at the top, as it can often be the most intimidating. Rather than starting off the top thinking you must make perfect turns from the get-go, find a way in, stop, take a couple of deep breaths, look around, and develop a plan for the next few turns.

If it's a mogul trail, search out the side of the trail where there are apt to be more rhythmic lines and rounder moguls, rather than the middle of the mogul trail which tends to be chaotic with choppy bumps and deep ruts. In this case, the strategy would be—don't ski the middle of the trail.

Now consider dropping into a steep chute—entering the slope tactically could determine the entire run. Often the lower entrance will avoid cornices, or maybe a rut that has formed. Or there might be an option of skiing along the ridge prior to dropping in, finding untracked snow, then maybe a traverse into the middle of the chute and through the gut. Here, the strategy would be finding the smoothest entrance, getting to the middle of the chute and chilling for a bit, then having a clear plan on how many turns you want to make and where you will stop.

Or how about glades. Rather than dropping right off the top and accelerating around a clump of trees, maybe there is a traverse to take into a small clearing. From there you can decide your line by looking for alleyways down the fall line that provide the best options and locations for stopping where needed.

In all these examples the key is to provide yourself the best chance for success by easing your way onto a slope or run, shaking off any tension, and developing a plan that works for you.

One of the most important tactics I teach is having a starting and stopping point, and breaking the mogul run, steep slope, or glades into sections. It is important not to be overly aggressive on the distance you ski. Remember, if you feel comfortable making three or four good solid turns and stopping, then do that. Most skiers get into trouble making too many turns, and have no idea what a good stopping point is—mainly, because they haven't thought about it.

By breaking the run into sections, you gain confidence in having a beginning and end to each section. Over time, as you get comfortable on a certain run, you can lengthen the distance you ski. It is always better to make four great turns, stop, and continue, than to blow the fifth turn, lose your balance, and fall on the sixth one.

Now consider the most important strategy of all: imperfection. Even the best of the best skiers can't make 100 percent perfect turns. I once asked a World Cup racer after they'd won a race how many perfect turns they'd made that day. They answered, "maybe 50 percent." Imagine that, if one of the best skiers in the world won a World Cup race with 50 percent perfect turns, us mere mortals are having the run of our lives if we're making 20 to 30 percent perfect turns.

In other words, lighten up on yourself. If you make a bad turn, don't let it contaminate the next good one. By adopting the strategy of imperfection and being less critical of your technique, over time you might start to enjoy the journey.

A Turning Ski is a Stable Ski

THERE HAS BEEN A BIG push in the last ten to fifteen years toward wider skis. "Fat skis" or "powder skis" have changed our perceptions of what skis should look like, because some have lost camber, some are flat with no camber, some have reverse camber, some have camber under the foot and tips and tails that turn up, or the so-called "early rise." All of this allows skiers of all abilities to explore more of the mountain because the ski glides on and through the snow more easily.

In the first edition of *All-Terrain Skiing*, published in 1996, I didn't address the changing landscape of ski design. Back then, shaped skis were just hitting the market and revolutionizing the industry. However, I wanted to focus my multimedia program (the book, video, and cards) on dynamic body motion, not equipment, and I still believe that should remain the focus for anyone looking to become an all-terrain skier.

Yet, today we are all skiing on wider skis, and the evolution of ski technology has expanded and enhanced our sport—there is no doubt about that. And overall, our turning radius has lengthened and become more directional, mainly because we are skiing *on* the snow, floating more than we did with straight skis.

However, wide skis of more than 88mm in width under your foot have significantly more surface area, and as a result don't track well in a straight line. Rather, they wobble in deep and cut-up snow, chatter and vibrate on hardpack and groomed snow. If you have ever felt your ski wobble under your foot while traversing or on the cat track, you know what I mean.

This has resulted in many skiers feeling like they are doing something wrong, but they are not—it's an equipment issue, not a performance issue. Here's the dilemma: the surface area of the ski, due to the increased width, causes the ski to scoot forward. This puts the feet of the skier in front of their hips, which puts them out of balance. The result is a lack of control, which is exhausting for the legs.

Let's talk about the length of the arc of a turn. The most stable part of skiing is the turn. If you want more stability with your wide skis, lengthen the arc and shorten the length of the transition between turns. After I make this statement in my camps and clinics, most skiers instantly think that a longer turn will mean going faster, resulting in acceleration they don't want. There is a slight increase in speed, however, you'll be more stable and confident. A stable ski is easier to control, and speed becomes less of an issue.

In general, when skiers turn to slow down, they make short turns and a long transition. The issue with this method is that they are spending more time standing on an unstable ski and a less time on a stable, turning ski. To gain stability, lengthen the arc of your turn and shorten the transition between your turn. So, if you have purchased fat skis to float over the snow and are then using them to make short turns, you are not gaining all the stability the ski is designed to provide.

Starting on a slope you are comfortable on, ski down the fall line. Tilt the ski on edge and let it find its designed arcing radius down the mountain. Be patient. Don't twist your feet, let the ski turn on its own. Keep your hands just below shoulder height and push them forward to keep your shoulders over your feet. As the skis come out of the turn, roll your feet quickly over to the new edge and let the skis arc down the fall line in the new turn.

Please note that I am talking about fall line skiing, not cross-hill skiing. Keep the ski in a long arcing turn in the fall line. You should be making a series of S turns that are long with short transitions, so the skis go from edge to edge. This will shorten the length of time the ski is flat and unstable.

You'll be amazed at how effortless it is to keep the skis turning under you in long stable turns. When we ski, we want to be efficient and intentional with our motion on the route down the mountain. Learning to stabilize these wider skis will result in more confidence and the time to have a nice long day mastering the mountain. When you add the slowing method of decelerating over a series of turns, allowing the skis to arc between them, you are experiencing an extremely rewarding level of mastery.

Searching for the Goods

ONE OF MY FAVORITE THINGS to do is listen to the lift line chatter on a powder day. There is an energy level that swells as skiers and riders roll into the queue in anticipation of the day ahead. The hardcore locals have the pole position in the front of the line, the diehard guests are in the second wave near the front, the wannabes who thought that fifteen minutes to opening would be early enough and the vacationers who wander in at nine are aghast at the length of the line.

Here are a few helpful hints while searching for powder:

Know your routes. I'm a big fan of repetition, and ski the same routes repeatedly. This pays off in many ways, like during and after storms. When you know the terrain you are lapping, it will also pay dividends and help you understand skier traffic and the patterns of where fresh windblown snow and powder is deposited.

Storm days are magic. These are the days you experience new snow overnight and then get to ski it the next day on the slopes. If you have done your homework, you will be ripping a line you know well in poor visibility and reaping the rewards of free refills along the way. The other advantage to skiing during the storm is shorter lift lines—as the storm builds during the day, the crowd dissipates, leaving the dedicated few to arc fresh turns till the "buzzer" goes off at 4 p.m.

If there has been a storm overnight and the "powder frenzy" is in full gear as the day breaks, have a plan and stick to it. Don't wait for others, and stay focused on the basics: where you'll park; what time you'll enter the lift line—these days it's an hour early or so mandatory for front-of-line access; dress for the wait; make friends in line; and, most of all, listen to the chatter—you'll glean a lot of intel on where to go and why.

I have a few hard and fast rules: never leave good snow to find better snow, and ski runs right off the lift, even if that means sacrificing vertical. Don't go from one lift line to another. Remember, while the cool kids are lining up for their dream Black Diamond run, you could be crushing powder in the trees, on wide-open trails, and in steep pitches holding deep powder pillows.

The day after the storm is often my favorite. The frenzy has dulled a bit, the glades are still holding pockets of fresh snowfall, and the mogul lines have filled in. However, the real magic for the day after the storm is locating where the wind transported the snow overnight. This is when your recon pays off—it could be the leeward side of a ridge, a vein of snow that develops in a gully, or a clearing in the woods. Knowing these stashes will dramatically expand your powder-to-turn, or PTT, ratio.

Now we turn to the calm after the storm, two or three days after the powder hounds have left, when the parking lots have empty spots. The lift lines are back to normal, the sun is shining, there is time for a proper cup of joe in the lodge, and your plan for the day is unfolding with a few close friends. Knowing the resort, your destination is the north by northeast, in search of cold, dry snow left unaffected by sun and tracks.

On these days, if you ride with the purpose and understanding that quality trumps quantity, you will be well rewarded for your efforts because the pitches still have pillows, the ruts are still soft, the bumps hold islands of snow, and in the woods, soft snow awaits above clumps of trees or just below them. As these kinds of powder days are often few and far between, it's always nice to maximize the ones we have while waiting for another yet to come.

A Lifetime Sentence

IT'S AN OLD JOKE, BUT one that rings true every time I hear it or tell it.

Question: Why are ski resorts like prison?

Answer: Because you do three to five months, for three to five years to life.

Well, I'm a lifer. My sentence started in 1983 at Magic Mountain, a small ski area in southern Vermont. I was the NASTAR guy—my tasks every Saturday and Sunday were to set the NASTAR racecourse, set the pace, sign up the competitors, and award the medals.

Since then, I've been transferred around the globe far and wide, from Val-d'Isère, France; Squaw Valley, California; Waterville Valley, New Hampshire; and Big Sky, Montana; to Valle Nevado, Chile.

One of my favorite musicians is John Eddie, who has a great song called "Forty." One of the verses goes like this:

"Well I'm a petered-out Peter Pan

Well sometimes I feel foolish I make my living singing in this band"

In other words, "when will he ever grow up?" I get asked that question a lot.

Years ago, I met the brother of a famous skier, who was attending Harvard. I asked him why he gave up skiing and if he ever wished he'd continued, based on his brother's success. His answer hit me like a ton of bricks. "When I realized skiing was just an extension of my adolescence, I had to give it up," he said.

I've pondered that answer for a long time now because, for me, skiing is also an extension of my own adolescence. I feel youthful every time I ski. The internal smile, the uncontrollable joy, and pleasure sliding over and through snow is magic—it never fails me.

I've also allowed my adolescent experiences to shape me. At sixteen, I had the opportunity to race a boat from Cape Cod, Massachusetts, to Bermuda. It was a hard trip, with big storms and lots of rain mixed with long periods of dead calm. The storms were so big that one boat sank during the race.

When we were safely on the dock, the navigator on our boat asked me what I thought of the trip, and I told him, "I loved it." He replied, "Really? You looked miserable much of the time!" I replied that that was how I knew I loved it—because I was willing to endure the hard parts.

Henry David Thoreau once said, "Truth and roses have thorns about them." That's how I feel about making my living as a ski bum. It's hard, *very* hard. I've paid a big price for this choice. I've almost died several times, and financially it might not have been the most stable of careers.

However, emotionally, spiritually, and physically, I can think of no other choice for my life. Skiing is my art form, my personal expression of life. It has provided me with an impressive canvas to teach and to be taught.

In Dan Millman's book *The Way of the Peaceful Warrior*, the main character asks his spiritual advisor how to find his way in life, and the advice given is: "You will fail many times, but in failing you will learn, and in learning you will find your way."

In the mountains I have been blessed to live multiple lifetimes, which has taught me to embrace my adolescence while being transformed by a life sentence of mountain living.

My wish for those of you who've experienced my All-Terrain Skiing program is that the magic of the mountains reveals itself to you, and you become an efficient lifelong skier who discovers the beauty of gliding on, over, and through the snow.

Ski for Life,
Dan Egan
2022

ACKNOWLEDGMENTS

IT IS NOT POSSIBLE TO recall the countless chairlift conversations and ski days as a ski student, racer, professional athlete, coach, and ski enthusiast. Together with family members, friends, colleagues, acquaintances, and strangers, I have had the pleasure of searching for the ultimate turn again and again around the globe. I love the passionate discussions, starting from the excitement of one day and ending with anticipation of the next. To me, that is where the inner science and soul of skiing exist off the mountain.

I wish to thank all six of my brothers and sisters: Mary Ellen, Bob, John, Sue, Ned, and Mike. We grew up skiing on hand-me-down equipment, and all of us are just a bit competitive, so life was a constant game of one-upmanship. The best part was having each other to ski with. We always had fun. A special thanks to my mother and father for having the patience and willingness to wake up and get us to the ski bus every Saturday, and especially for allowing me to choose my career in skiing. This book is dedicated to them, Marlen and Robert. They have both since passed, and I miss them each and every day.

Regarding specific ideas and concepts, I would like to thank the following people for their contributions: John Egan, Mike Egan, Ken Scott, Ben Brosseau, Chris Jones, Tim Mitchell, Weems Westfeldt, Ken Marisseau, Henry Schniewind, Marty Heckelman, Mike Wenner, Stephen Kassin, Mike Calley, Mike Ewing, Dean Decas, Ed Brennan, Lizzy Day, Tom Day, Hank de'Vre, Eric and Rob DesLauriers, Eric Foch, Tom Grissom, Warren Miller, Marcus Caston, Dennis Ouellette, Glen Parkinson, Doug Pfieffer, David Seymore, all my past clients from the Extreme Team Advanced Ski Clinics, and current clients of Skiclinics.com. Over the last thirty or so years it has been an amazing experience, skiing the across North America, Europe, and South America with you all.

The App for this project was developed by Jasper Lapkin, a young creative developer living in the heart of the Wasatch Mountains of Utah. I'm grateful to his insight and ease of programming for this project.

In January of 2022, we traveled to Laax, Switzerland—the perfect spot for shooting much of the video needed for this project. In a week, Patti Johnson recorded the majority of video footage for the thirty-one drills and skills outlined in this program. Her patience, practicality, and attention to detail is a constant blessing for me, both on and off the slopes. Skiing around Laax was amazing; the wide open terrain, matched by the long vertical, provided the variety needed, all set among the backdrop of the Swiss Alps.

In putting this book together, I owe a great big Thank You to Jack B. Rochester, who has provided guidance, wisdom, and the right words time and time again, and to Caitlin M. Park and Kristin Thornburgh, Jack's editorial associates at Joshua Tree Interactive. My appreciation goes to Sammy Blair, who handles all things from marketing, scheduling, PR, and so much more. To Kathryn Costello, our webmaster. Additional video was captured by Tom Day, from Warren Miller's Future Retro film, and Steep Productions, owned and operated by Satchel Burns. When it comes to ski industry friends and mentors, for constant guidance and wisdom, thank you to the following individuals: Marty and Shelagh Riehs, Matt Beck, Bernie Weichsel, Billy Fallon, Dan Cooney, Noel Lyons, Pam Fletcher, Gary Nate, Phil and Trish Pugliese, Andy Sainsbury, Mike Ewing, Paul Mannelin, Ken Scott, Christine Baker, Stacey Mesuda, Gary Miller, Mike Specian, and Clara Greb.

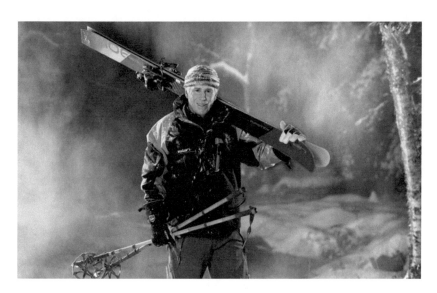

ABOUT THE AUTHOR

DAN EGAN IS A WORLD-RENOWNED skier and pioneer of extreme sports. He has appeared in thirteen Warren Miller ski films and is known for skiing the most remote regions of the world with his brother, John Egan. In 2001, *Powder* magazine named him one of the most influential skiers of our time, and in 2016 he was inducted into the US Skiing & Snowboarding Hall of Fame.

During the late 1980s and 1990s, Dan Egan's skiing exploits mirrored and chronicled the geopolitical landscape of the world, an approach that played a critical role in redefining the *extreme* in extreme sports. His innovative adventures exceeded the extreme physical challenge of the mountains and forced ski bums and civilians alike to see skiing (and sports in general) as a means of engaging with the cultures, histories, and diverse people of the world. Dan's global approach to extreme sports created the foundation for massive growth in international travel and the demand for technology to capture and share individuals' adventures and experiences while abroad. As a ski ambassador, coach, and guide, he can be found on the snow in Waterville Valley, New Hampshire; Big Sky, Montana; Valle Nevado, Chile; Val-d'Isère France; and across the Alps, sharing his knowledge and passion for the sport. He is sponsored by Leki, Big Sky, Elan, and Alps & Meters.

Dan has authored four books, *All-Terrain Skiing*, *All-Terrain Skiing II*, *Courage to Persevere* (co-authored with Bill Fallon), and his latest book, *Thirty Years in a White Haze* (co-authored with Eric Wilbur). Keep an eye out for Egan's soon to be released new book, *Mastering the Skiing Mind*. For more information, visit his website dan-egan.com.

For more information about Dan Egan: www.Dan-Egan.com

To Ski with Dan, go to: www.SkiClinics.com

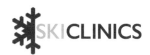

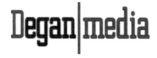

Made in the USA
Columbia, SC
18 October 2024

44659103R00065